Medical Scribe Training Manual

MedChart Medical Scribes, LLC

TABLE OF CONTENTS

1

INTRODUCTION

With the creation of Electronic Medical Records (EMRs), medical scribes are becoming more prevalent in the medical. A medical scribe is a documentation specialist who is trained on the basics of completing a medical chart in the EMR. The medical scribe will stand in the background of the examination room and take notes during the medical interview, allowing the Physician to place focus directly on the patient. They also retrieve lab results, know emergency room coding basics, and are considered an "extra set of eyes and ears" for the Physicians, among other duties. A successful medical scribe program will increase patient satisfaction scores, increase Physician job satisfaction, increase productivity, increase the net revenue of the emergency department, and decrease the emergency room waiting time.

Whether you are an emergency department administrator learning to run your medical scribe program or you are a future medical scribe, you will find this manual to be a valuable tool as you train others to become a medical scribe, or as you become a medical scribe yourself! Regardless, you are now an important part of the emergency department team where you will be directly responsible increasing efficiency within the department. Each emergency department location will offer a unique experience and will ultimately give the scribe an in-depth experience in the medical field as they prepare for a career in medicine. For administrators, your emergency department will reap the benefits of a medical scribe program and Physicians will seek out your ER as a preferred destination to practice medicine.

As a medical scribe, you will be working alongside Physicians and documenting their encounters with patients on the electronic medical record system. In addition to this, your responsibilities include, but are not limited to:

- Documenting the entire interaction between the patient and the physician
- Working as a liaison between the physician and other ED staff
- Alerting the physician if a chart is incomplete
- Keeping a an up to date record of the status of patients being seen in the emergency department to facilitate efficient dispositions
- Keeping your physician informed as test results become available
- Ensuring proper documentation requirements are met

Your position as a scribe will be a valuable first step in your pursuit of a career in medicine. You will gain experience in an emergency department where you will work alongside the physicians and interact with various members of the healthcare team. As you progress you will begin to anticipate what tests will be ordered based on a patient's clinical presentation and will learn to interpret the results of these tests. You will have extensive training and experience in writing a medical chart, which will give you an advantage in Medical School, Physician Assistant School, or Nursing School. In addition, the physicians you work with will be valuable resources for you in obtaining letters of recommendation. As a scribe, we expect you to treat your position with the highest level of professionalism and respect.

Good luck!

Christopher Anderson, MBA, MS
President at MedChart Medical Scribes, LLC

2

MEDCHART MEDICAL SCRIBE POLICIES

Attitude

As a medical scribe, it is important to have respect for all individuals you encounter in the emergency department including all staff, patients, and visitors. As a MedChart Medical Scribe you are expected to demonstrate a high level of professionalism. We expect our employees to not only exhibit a professional demeanor, but also maintain a friendly, courteous and positive attitude in every situation.

Service

MedChart Medical Scribes guarantees highly motivated and dependable medical scribes to all of the medical communities we serve. It is essential that the physicians we work with receive a well trained and knowledgeable scribe for each shift. During your time as a scribe you should constantly strive for self-improvement. As an aspiring health care student, your time spent as a scribe will hopefully be a life-changing and enlightening experience. At MedChart, we are dedicated to the continued education of our scribes in order to maintain a high standard of excellence.

 Over the course of the first 90 days of employment, you will go through a rigorous training process to assure that you are well equipped with the necessary information to succeed as a scribe. After the initial training period, you will periodically be assessed throughout your employment with MedChart to ensure that each medical chart fulfills our high standards.

Dress Code

You must wear scrubs issued to you by MedChart Medical Scribes. You may not wear any other color scrubs, as this will create confusion to patients and employees in the emergency department. Your scrubs must be clean and should not be altered in any way. Undergarments should never be visible. You must wear closed-toe shoes, and we recommend they be comfortable as you will be on your feet for the majority of the shift. No sweatshirts, jackets, fleeces, or sweaters are permitted in the ED. However, you may purchase a matching scrub jacket or wear a solid colored shirt under your scrubs (may not be a fleece or sweatshirt material). No visible body piercings or tattoos are allowed. Make-up, nail color, and hairstyles should be professional in appearance and appropriate for a medical setting. Violation of any of the above policies will result in your removal from the medical facility, which will be counted as an absence in your file.

Zero Tolerance Drug and Alcohol Policy

MedChart Medical Scribes has a zero tolerance drug and alcohol policy. The use of any illicit drugs while employed by MedChart is strictly prohibited; this includes prescription drugs that you do not have a prescription for. We reserve the right to test any employee at any time for the presence of drugs in their system if suspicion arises. Any positive findings on such a screening will result in immediate termination. In addition, being under the influence of alcohol during your shift will result in immediate termination.

Safety

As a scribe, you are strictly prohibited from any direct patient contact. However, you will be working in an emergency department where you may be exposed to various illnesses and hazards. We ask that you take all necessary precautions while working in the ED to ensure your personal health and safety. Such safety measures include but are not limited to:
- Never touch anything that has any blood or bodily fluids on it, or that has been in contact with blood or bodily fluids.
- You are allowed to open sterile packages, but never "glove up" or assist in any patient care.
- Do not handle any needles or sharps.
- Take all precautions when entering a room with an infectious patient including wearing a mask or gown if required.
- If an x-ray is being done in a room, exit the room to avoid radiation exposure.
- Do not assist in restraining any patients.
- If you feel threatened in any way by a patient or visitor, alert the necessary personnel such as the charge nurse or security.

At MedChart Medical Scribes, we will require all of our scribes to be up to date in immunizations and vaccinations as required by the given department. These specific requirements will be relayed to you depending on the facility you are working in.

If you ever feel that your own personal safety is threatened, do not hesitate to contact the appropriate personnel whether it is employee health or the ED's security staff. Always report any incidents to MedChart Medical Scribes.

Attendance Policy

Scribes are expected to be on time for each scheduled shift. This means being ready to see patients with your physician when the shift begins. Therefore, we request that you arrive 10 minutes before the shift start time in order to allow adequate time to clock in, greet your physician and prepare yourself to scribe. Clocking in after your scheduled start time will result in a tardy and will be noted in your disciplinary file. An accumulation of 3 tardies within a 6-month period will result in a review of your file and possible termination. Each physician is assigned one scribe for each shift. Therefore, it is your responsibility to attend your shift, or find appropriate coverage should an unforeseen event arise. We do not allow you to "call in sick," and should you become ill it is your responsibility to find shift coverage. In the case of an emergency such as a death in your family or hospitalization you should immediately contact your Chief Scribe or Chris Anderson at 248-925-8907. You will be required to provide sufficient documentation as proof of your emergency. MedChart takes absences very seriously and any absence will result in review of the scribe's disciplinary file and could result in immediate termination.

It is never acceptable to ask your physician for time off or for permission to arrive late or leave early. The ED is unpredictable and therefore there may be times when your shift time ends despite there still being open patient charts. In this event you must finish all charts and are not permitted to leave until the physician gives you permission. We ask that you always remain flexible and willing to help out. Should a scribe fail to show up for the shift after yours, offer to stay and help the next physician until another scribe arrives. In the event that this occurs, call your chief scribe or any member of the MedChart corporate staff and they will take steps to have another scribe come in to work.

You are an employee of MedChart Medical Scribes, and as such, all absences or schedule changes must be approved through us. Any scribe that fails to show up for a shift without contacting management will be subject to immediate termination. In the event of inclement weather, you are expected to attend your shift unless contacted by your trainer scribe or an executive member of MedChart's staff. If you have any questions or concerns regarding the attendance policy, contact your supervisor.

Meal Breaks

You are expected to see all patients with your physician, there are no scheduled meal breaks. The physician may take a short meal break, at which time you will be allowed to take a break. You should be prepared to bring a lunch or snacks as there will not be enough time to leave the hospital for food. Under no circumstances are you allowed to ask your physician for an extended break. However, if your physician decides not to take a break at all, you may ask to take a short break to eat. Please be considerate of your physician in this case, and be sure that there are no patients waiting to be seen. In addition, please be respectful of all ED rules and only have food in designated areas.

Cell Phone Use

Cell phone use is strictly prohibited in the ED. Personal calls, instant messaging, social networking, and/or texting are not allowed. Your cell phone should not be on you while you are working. Not only will this keep you free from distraction, it will allow you to provide the highest level of service to your physician and preserve the privacy of the patients. If for any reason you need to make a phone call, you may take a short break and step outside the department at a time when your physician does not need you.

Behavior in the Emergency Department

While working in the emergency department, patient volume varies and there may be times that are slower than others. Therefore, you are permitted to bring homework or reading material with you to your shift. However, this should never interfere in any way with your role as a scribe. If an issue arises where personal materials distract a scribe, he or she will lose the privilege of bringing these materials to the ED. Please limit all Internet use to work related searches such as the spelling of a medication or unknown medical term. Accessing social networking sites or browsing the web for entertainment is not permitted. As a MedChart Medical Scribe you are expected to act as a professional. If any physician complaint arises about a scribe not being focused on his or her responsibilities, it will be noted in the scribe's disciplinary file. Multiple offenses may result in the scribe's employment termination.

Social Networking Policy

While it is understood that scribes may use social networking sites outside of work, it is important to maintain professionalism. As a member of the medical community you should be mindful of what you are sharing online. Posting any information about what you may see or hear in the ED not only results in immediate termination but is also a violation of HIPPA and is punishable by law. You may not make any mention of any patient or encounter in the ED, even if you consider it to be public information. HIPAA laws are very serious and should not be taken lightly.

Furthermore, use common sense when posting anything on the Internet. Consider whether the content you are posting is appropriate in a professional setting, especially as a future medical professional. You are representing yourself and any negative online content may also be a deterrent to future admissions committees.

The History of the Medical Scribe

There are various dates as to when the medical scribe first appeared in emergency medicine. In 1999, the Advisory Board Company published a capsule titled "Charting Scribe" and reviewed the practice of using a medical scribe in emergency medicine. The Advisory Board Company assigned the practice of using a charting scribe with a Clinical Initiatives Center Grade of "A–." Furthermore, the charting scribe was "strongly recommended for most members, a highly effective practice for reducing ED LOS and improving patient satisfaction."[1]

While medical scribes programs were scarcely used in the emergency room setting, it wasn't until the U.S. Congress pushed for the implementation of Electronic Medical Records that resulted in the need for medical scribes. The American Recovery and Reinvestment Act of 2009 provided incentives and penalties to entice physicians and hospital systems to adopt EMRs. As current legislation stands, all medical records must be transitioned to Electronic Medical Records by the end of 2014. Suddenly, new EMRs began appearing as the opportunity for profits arose. With large hospital systems integrating new EMRs, many physicians did not like the fact that they had to change their ways – they were being forced to put a patient's medical record on a computer, or pay a penalty. With the U.S.'s aging physician base and steady increase in hospital visits by the newer senior citizen class of 'baby-boomers,' there were immediate and substantial drops in productivity and efficiency. The emergency room is a very busy department of the hospital and a drop in productivity has a chain reaction leading to decreased patient satisfaction scores, decreased chart reimbursement amounts, and decreased general

---

[1] Advisory Board Company, The. (1999). Practice #3: Charting Scribe. Liberating Physician Time , 59-81.

profitability of the emergency room as a whole. Studies show that there is a 30% drop in productivity directly correlated to the implementation of a new EMR. Even after the hospital staff becomes accustomed to the new computerized medical records and changes in processes, emergency rooms were still unable to attain efficiency levels from before the EMR was implemented.

Emergency rooms had to account for this drop in productivity and focus on revenue-generating opportunities. A medical scribe program has shown to not only get the emergency room profits and patient satisfaction levels back to the pre-EMR levels, but an increase of 10% beyond the initial levels. With the implementation of a medical scribe program, the emergency room will see an increase in chart reimbursement, an increase in patient satisfaction and physician satisfaction scores, an increase in net revenue.

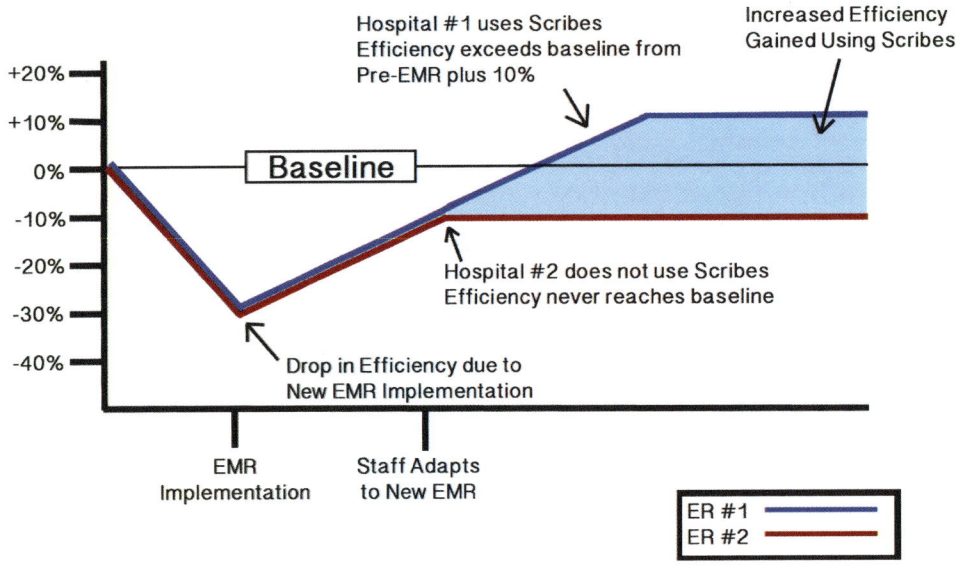

It is a sure bet that the Physician did not go to medical school to update computer medical charts – they chose to be a Physician to help people and make decisions in the best interests of their patients. To adequately utilize the Emergency Center Physician (ECP), they should be in and out of patient examination rooms to keep the patient flow steady. It should be the goal of the hospital to effectively use its most expensive asset, the Physicians. Medical scribes assist the physicians with the clerical duties of emergency medicine and they are a less expensive option than having the physician stay after hours to complete documentation.

The Functions of a Medical Scribe

Medical scribes will work alongside the physicians and provide them with any assistance they may need. Each physician can choose how he or she would like to work with a scribe, but research shows scribes are most useful while:

- Assuming a majority of patient documentation as the scribe records the interaction between the physician and patient
- Tracking patient orders and alerting the physician as results become available
- Working as a liaison between the physician and other hospital staff members as needed
- Ensuring all charts are complete and contain the correct amount of elements for billing purposes
- Assisting patients with any non-medical needs
- Taking and making phone calls for the physician
- Completing discharge and follow up instructions for patients who are discharged

Guidelines for Program Success for the ECP

In order for the medical scribe program to be a success, the Physicians must also be prepared to change the way they document the chart. Using the acronym, SCRIBE, there are guidelines that should be set for the ECP to increase the value of the medical scribe to the department. Medical scribes are in the emergency department to help the Physician's workload; they are there to make your life easier.

S – **Share**
C – **Create**
R – **Record**
I – **Inform**
B – **Build**
E – **Evaluate**

SHARE the way the physician prefers documenting the patient interaction. Medical scribes are trained on creating a medical chart, but each physician has his/her preferences on how a chart is completed. By communicating this to the scribe before the shift begins, the Physician will save time by not editing the scribe's note.

CREATE a user-friendly dialogue between the patient and the ECP. The medical scribe is in the background completing the medical chart and the Physician should get as much information as possible for the chart. Use open-ended questions like, "What brings you in today?" or "Tell me more about…"

RECORD other useful information that the scribe has not yet entered into the medical chart and enter CPOE.

INFORM the medical scribe of the specific tests you are waiting for and any special directions regarding certain patients.

BUILD a rapport with the medical scribe. At one point in your career, you have been in the position that the medical scribe is in. The scribes are a sponge as they soak up all of the information you give them.

EVALUATE the scribes through a company evaluation form and point out the areas for the scribe to improve. Also, please note areas where the scribe is excelling.

Template for ECP / Scribe Interaction

Event	ECP	Scribe
1. Pre-Patient Discussion	Emergency Center Physicians (ECP) need to complete macros for review of systems and physical examinations for minimally male, female, pediatric and adult patients. Prior to commencing the shift, these macros need to be shared with the scribes. Emergency Physicians need to inform the scribe on how they like to document their decision-making; either the ECP types or scribe types it. The ECP needs to tell the scribe how they like the note done whether it is via Note writer or free text for the HPI. Emergency Physicians need to empty their inboxes.	Scribes can assist the ECP's with the building of those macros and sharing them. Scribes can assist the ECP's in emptying their inboxes.
2. Patient Interaction	Emergency Physicians need to interview the patient in a fashion that allows the scribe to create a viable HPI. The story should begin with the chief complaint, "What brought you in today?" **History & Physical Examination** Utilize the scribe as an extension of the computer/dictation. Need to create and tell a logical story. Emergency Physicians can document by	Scribe will use the answer to that question as their chief complaint. Scribe transcribes the story heard from the physician and family responses. Scribes can delete past history

	exception assuming that the scribe is aware of their normal template for review of systems and physical examination.	non-pertinent negative information.
	Review of Systems is generated by the physician. Many of these fields can be prompted by simple questions, i.e., if you ask the patient if they are having any pain and they answer no, the prepopulated review of systems pain related issues can be addressed almost immediately.	Scribes access templates and assumes organ systems not discussed are normal.
	Physical Examination Physicians should convey to the scribes the pertinent positives or essentially what is not on their templates as the templates should all be constructed to reflect essentially a normal physical exam. The pertinent positives should be deviations from that normal physical exam.	
	Differential Diagnosis The differential diagnosis should be discussed with the family.	Scribe listens for differential diagnosis and discussion with the family and transcribes minimally two differential diagnoses.
3. Post-Patient Interaction	ECP completes the CPOE.	Scribe completes the note.
4. Ongoing Visit	ECP conveys to the scribe the essence of	Scribe documents ongoing

Documentation	the phone call for documentation purposes.	phone calls and contents of those phone calls and strategies.
5. Discharge	The ECP reviews the shared chart for final approval.	Scribes have completed their note including specific billing documentation regarding EKG, rhythm strip interpretation, pulse oximetry and critical care coding. The scribe then shares the note with the emergency physician.
6. After ECP Stops Seeing Patients for Shift	All notes must be signed.	Scribes check the ECP box to insure that all inboxes are empty.

Other fundamental tenants:

1. The scribe keeps pace with the emergency physician. The ECP should not be waiting for the scribe to complete documentation prior to moving on.
2. The HPI and ROS should be completed 90% in the room
3. The PEx can be started in the room and sometimes finished depending on the patient.
4. The PEx can also be completed after orders are done or later on when there is downtime.

3

HIPAA COMPLIANCE

HIPAA, the Health Insurance Portability and Accountability Act of 1996, is a law passed that provides regulations regarding use and disclosure of health records. Also known as the Privacy Rule, HIPAA defines how "covered entities", or anyone with access to an individual's health records, can use an individual's personal health information (PHI). The Privacy Rule does understand that some health information must be shared in order to promote high quality healthcare. Therefore, it allows for sharing of information while protecting an individual's identity. The following is a brief overview of HIPAA.

Overview of the Privacy Rule

The following is a list of guidelines set forth by HIPAA:
1. Patients have control over the use of their PHI, which includes any personal identification information (name, birth date, MRN) that may link them to health records.
2. HIPPA sets boundaries for use and disclosure of health records, including "minimum use". This means that a person with access to an individual's health record may only access the minimum amount of information necessary to complete the task at hand.
3. Establishes national standards which healthcare providers must adhere to.
4. Limits use of PHI in order to minimize chance of inappropriate disclosure.
5. Enforces strict compliance with all privacy measures and holds violators legally accountable with civil or criminal penalties.

Who Can Access PHI?

Anyone in the ED has access to information about the patients. This includes physicians, clerks, nurses, volunteers, and scribes.

What Should You Do?

When working in the ED, you notice your neighbor's name on the board and see that she is there for chest pain. She is close friends with your mom and you know that your mom would want to know that her friend is in the hospital. What should you do?

A. When you get home from your shift, call your mom to tell her you saw her friend. They are friends so the woman will probably want your mom to know she was there.

B. Keep the information to yourself. If this woman wants her friends to know she is in the ED she can tell them herself, otherwise it is a violation of her privacy to disclose this information.

C. Wait a few weeks and then mention the event to your mom. Since the woman is already out of the hospital it doesn't matter if you share this information.

Correct answer: B. Treat EVERY patient with the same respect and privacy. It doesn't matter if you think this is common knowledge.

A trauma case comes into the ED and a resident sees the patient. You overhear that the patient has some severe injuries, but not what they are. Should you...

A. Look at the results of the radiology. Everyone is talking about the patient anyway, its basically public information.

B. Look at the X-ray results that the resident left up on the screen. Its not like you are accessing the information on your own.

C. Leave the chart alone. This is not a patient you are seeing, therefore it is outside your job responsibility.

Correct answer: C.
A is incorrect; this is NOT public information. Others should not be talking about the patient in public areas.
B is incorrect; the resident should not have left these results on the screen, this in itself is a violation of HIPAA.

Your grandmother was admitted to the hospital yesterday. You haven't heard any updates on her status yet. What should you do?

A. Since you have access to the hospital's medical records, you open your grandmother's chart. She is your family member so you are not violating privacy.

B.	You wait until your break and call a family member to see if there are any updates. Looking at her records is outside of your job and therefore should not be opened.

C.	I can look at her labs as long as I don't open up the note.

Correct answer: B. You may not access ANY chart that is not a necessary part of your job, this includes family members. Labs are also included in PHI and should not be opened by you.

HIPAA violations are not tolerated in the health care industry and any HIPAA violation will lead to your dismissal from your medical scribe company, including MedChart Medical Scribes, LLC. MedChart Medical Scribes, LLC will not defend any of its employees who violate the HIPAA laws at any time. This text is only for informational purposes only and all official questions and rulings should be directed to the U.S. Department of Health and Human Services directly.

The next three pages are taken directly from the U.S. Department of Health and Human Services website at http://www.hhs.gov/ocr/privacy.[2]

The Standards for Privacy of Individually Identifiable Health Information ("Privacy Rule") establishes, for the first time, a set of national standards for the protection of certain health information. The U.S. Department of Health and Human Services ("HHS") issued the Privacy Rule to implement the requirement of the Health Insurance Portability and Accountability Act of 1996 ("HIPAA").

The Privacy Rule standards address the use and disclosure of individuals' health information—called "protected health information" by organizations subject to the Privacy Rule — called "covered entities," as well as standards for individuals' privacy rights to understand and control how their health information is used. Within HHS, the Office for Civil Rights ("OCR") has responsibility for implementing and enforcing the Privacy Rule with respect to voluntary compliance activities and civil money penalties. A major goal of the Privacy Rule is to assure that individuals' health information is properly protected while allowing the flow of health information needed to provide and promote high quality health care and to protect the public's health and well being. The Rule strikes a balance that permits important uses of information, while protecting the privacy of people who seek care and healing.

---

[2] U.S. Department of Health and Human Services. (2012). Health Information Privacy. Retrieved 01 15, 2012, from U.S. Department of Health and Human Services: http://www.hhs.gov/ocr/privacy/

Given that the health care marketplace is diverse, the Rule is designed to be flexible and comprehensive to cover the variety of uses and disclosures that need to be addressed.

This is a summary of key elements of the Privacy Rule and not a complete or comprehensive guide to compliance. Entities regulated by the Rule are obligated to comply with all of its applicable requirements and should not rely on this summary as a source of legal information or advice. To make it easier for entities to review the complete requirements of the Rule, provisions of the Rule referenced in this summary are cited in notes at the end of this document. To view the entire Rule, and for other additional helpful information about how it applies, see the OCR website: http://www.hhs.gov/ocr/hipaa. In the event of a conflict between this summary and the Rule, the Rule governs.

The Privacy Rule protects all "individually identifiable health information" held or transmitted by a covered entity or its business associate, in any form or media, whether electronic, paper, or oral. The Privacy Rule calls this information "protected health information (PHI). "Individually identifiable health information" is information, including demographic data, that relates to: the individual's past, present or future physical or mental health or condition, the provision of health care to the individual, or the past, present, or future payment for the provision of health care to the individual, and that identifies the individual or for which there is a reasonable basis to believe can be used to identify the individual. Individually identifiable health information includes many common identifiers (e.g., name, address, birth date, Social Security Number).

A major purpose of the Privacy Rule is to define and limit the circumstances in which an individual's protected heath information may be used or disclosed by covered entities. The Privacy Rule requires a covered entity to treat a "personal representative" the same as the individual, with respect to uses and disclosures of the individual's protected health information, as well as the individual's rights under the Rule.

A personal representative is a person legally authorized to make health care decisions on an individual's behalf or to act for a deceased individual or the estate. The Privacy Rule permits an exception when a covered entity has a reasonable belief that the personal representative may be abusing or neglecting the individual, or that treating the person as the personal representative could otherwise endanger the individual.

The Rule provides processes for persons to file complaints with HHS, describes the responsibilities of covered entities to provide records and compliance reports and to cooperate with, and permit access to information for, investigations and compliance reviews.

Civil Money Penalties

HHS may impose civil money penalties on a covered entity of $100 per failure to comply with a Privacy Rule requirement. That penalty may not exceed $25,000 per year for multiple violations of the identical Privacy Rule requirement in a calendar year.

Criminal Penalties

A person who knowingly obtains or discloses individually identifiable health information in violation of HIPAA faces a fine of $50,000 and up to one-year imprisonment.

The criminal penalties increase to $100,000 and up to five years imprisonment if the wrongful conduct involves false pretenses, and to $250,000 and up to ten years imprisonment if the wrongful conduct involves the intent to sell, transfer, or use individually identifiable health information for commercial advantage, personal gain, or malicious harm. Criminal sanctions will be enforced by the Department of Justice.

4

CMS CORE MEASURES AND PQRI

The Joint Commission

Hospitals are accredited by a safety and quality evaluation given by the Joint Commission, formerly known as JCAHO. Every 2-3 years, hospitals are re-evaluated, meaning you may be working in the emergency department while the Joint Commission is there. Passing these inspections is absolutely vital for hospital administration and the emergency room staff in order to continue to receive Medicare reimbursement. There are specific core measures that involve emergency physicians, which are updated frequently. Each core measure involves a detailed list of procedures that each member of the department must follow. The emergency physician is responsible for some of these actions and as a scribe, your job is to document that they are completed. It is of the upmost importance to correctly document all care given by your physician, and ensure all core measures are met and properly documented.

Currently, of the eleven core measure sets, there are only two situations in which the core measures affect the emergency department – Pneumonia and Acute Myocardial Infarction (AMI). For more information on core measure sets, visit The Joint Commission's website at http://www.jointcommission.org. The core measure sets below were produced from The Joint Commission's website [3]:

> *Set Measure ID: PN-3a*
>
> *Performance Measure Name: Blood Cultures Performed Within 24 Hours Prior to or 24 Hours After Hospital Arrival for Patients Who Were Transferred or Admitted to the ICU Within 24 Hours of Hospital Arrival*
>
> *Description: Pneumonia patients transferred or admitted to the ICU within 24 hours of hospital arrival, who had blood cultures performed within 24 hours prior to or 24 hours after hospital arrival.*

---

[3] Joint Commission, The. (2010, 10 22). Core Measure Sets. Retreived 01 15, 2012, from The Joint Commission: http://www.jointcommission.org/core_measure_set/

Rationale: Published pneumonia treatment guidelines from ATS/IDSA recommend performance of blood cultures for all inpatients with severe pneumonia to optimize therapy. Improved survival has been associated with optimal therapy. In addition, the yield of clinically useful information is greater if the culture is collected before antibiotics are administered. The actual performance of a culture has been added to this measure because restricting measurement to culture collection prior to antibiotics provides an incentive for hospitals not to perform a culture in any patient who has already received antibiotics.

Set Measure ID: PN-3b

Performance Measure Name: *Blood Cultures Performed in the Emergency Department Prior to Initial Antibiotic Received in Hospital*

Description: *Pneumonia patients whose initial emergency room blood culture specimen was collected prior to first hospital dose of antibiotics. This measure focuses on the treatment provided to Emergency Department patients prior to admission orders.*

Rationale: *Published pneumonia treatment guidelines recommend performance of blood cultures for all inpatients to optimize therapy. Improved survival has been associated with optimal therapy. In addition, the yield of clinically useful information is greater if the culture is collected before antibiotics are administered.*

Set Measure ID: PN-6

Performance Measure Name: *Initial Antibiotic Selection for Community-Acquired Pneumonia (CAP) in Immunocompetent Patients*

PN-6b: Initial Antibiotic Selection for Community-Acquired Pneumonia (CAP) in Immunocompetent Patients – Non ICU Patients

PN-6a: Initial Antibiotic Selection for Community-Acquired Pneumonia (CAP) in Immunocompetent Patients – Intensive Care Unit (ICU) Patients

Description: *Immunocompetent patients with Community-Acquired Pneumonia who receive an initial antibiotic regimen during the first 24 hours that is consistent with current guidelines.*

Note: *CMS data is transmitted as patient level data while the Joint Commission's data is transmitted as aggregate level data. Therefore, in order for The Joint Commission to distinguish between ICU and non-ICU patients, two separate measures (PN-6a and PN-6b) are required for data transmission.*

Rationale: *The current North American antibiotic guidelines for Community-Acquired Pneumonia in immunocompetent patients are from the Centers for Disease Control and Prevention (CDC), the Infectious Diseases Society of America (IDSA), the Canadian Infectious Disease Society / Canadian Thoracic Society (CIDS/CTS), and the American Thoracic Society (ATS). All four reflect that Streptococcus pneumoniae is the most common cause of CAP, that treatment that covers "atypical" pathogens (e.g., Legionella species, Chlamydia pneumoniae, Mycoplasma pneumoniae) can be associated with improved survival, and that the prevalence of antibiotic resistant S. pneumoniae is increasing.*

Set Measure ID #: AMI-1

Performance Measure Name: *Aspirin at Arrival*
Description: *Acute myocardial infarction (AMI) patients who received aspirin within 24 hours before or after hospital arrival*

Rationale: The early use of aspirin in patients with acute myocardial infarction results in a significant reduction in adverse events and subsequent mortality. The benefits of aspirin therapy on mortality are comparable to fibrinolytic therapy. The combination of aspirin and fibrinolytics provides additive benefits for patients with ST-elevation myocardial infarction (ISIS-2, 1988). Aspirin is also effective in patients with non-ST-elevation myocardial infarction (Theroux, 1988 and RISC Group, 1990). National guidelines strongly recommend early aspirin for patients hospitalized with AMI (Antman, 2004; Antman, 2008; and Anderson, 2007).

Physician Quality Reporting Initiative

The Physician Quality Reporting Initiative (PQRI) was formally launched under a provision of the Tax Relief and Health Care Act of 2006. In 2011, the program name was changed to Physician Quality Reporting System (PQRS). The following italicized content explains PQRI and does into further detail about its measures. This information can be found on the American College of Emergency Physicians website[4].

The PQRS program provides a financial incentive to eligible professionals for voluntarily reporting data on specific quality measures applied to the Medicare population. Medicare Part C–Medicare Advantage beneficiaries are not included in this program. Under PQRS, incentives will be paid simply for satisfactorily reporting on designated quality measures. However, it is anticipated that PQRS eventually will be transitioned to a formal pay for performance model. CMS uses the word "report" to mean a claim form where the medical services reported (CPT codes and ICD-9 codes) indicate an opportunity for PQRS measure reporting. The 16 individual measures that pertain to emergency medicine are available for submission by a claim form or a qualified registry.

---

[4] American College of Emergency Physicians. (2012). Physician Quality Reporting System   FAQ. Retrieved 01 15, 2012, from the American College of Emergency Physicians: http://www.acep.org/content.aspx?id=30492

PQRS measures are available to indicate that the measure was performed, or not performed based on an acceptable exemption or exclusion. If a specific PQRS code is not submitted, the opportunity to receive the financial incentive is forfeited.

The 2012 PQRS System Measures List identifies over 300 quality measures. There are 4 new measures that apply to Emergency Medicine for 2012.

As required by applicable statutes, the list for each year is developed through formal notice-and-comment rulemaking in the previous year.

Incentive payments are available until 2014. Beginning in 2015, physicians who do not satisfactorily report PQRS measures will be subject to negative payment adjustments. Incentive payments and negative payment adjustments are based upon the physician's total allowable Medicare charges for a given year. The program applies to physicians as well as Physician Assistants and Nurse Practitioners who report on eligible services provided to Medicare beneficiaries. Credit for quality measures will be assigned to the reporting provider, based on his or her individual National Provider Identifier (NPI); however, payment of the bonus will be based on the Taxpayer Identification Number (TIN) of the reporting entity.

What Quality Measures are Applicable to Emergency Medicine for 2012?

For 2012, there are 4 new measures now totaling 16 potentially linked to emergency medicine by CPT E/M codes 99281 through 99285 and/or critical care services (CPT codes 99291), as well as specific ICD-9 diagnosis codes.

Measure #28 Aspirin at Arrival for Acute Myocardial Infarction (AMI)
Percentage of patients with an emergency department discharge diagnosis of AMI who had documentation of receiving aspirin within 24 hours before emergency department arrival or during emergency department stay

Measure #31 Stroke and Stroke Rehabilitation: Deep Vein Thrombosis Prophylaxis (DVT) for Ischemic Stroke or Intracranial Hemorrhage (only critical care code 99291 applies)

Percentage of patients aged 18 years and older with a diagnosis of ischemic stroke or intracranial hemorrhage who received DVT prophylaxis by end of hospital day two. Though the specifications further state: "It is anticipated that clinicians who care for patients with a diagnosis of ischemic stroke or intracranial hemorrhage in the hospital setting will submit this measure," making these measures less applicable to Emergency Physicians in the acute care setting.

Measure #54 Electrocardiogram Performed for Non-Traumatic Chest Pain

Percentage of patients aged 40 years and older with an emergency department discharge diagnosis of non-traumatic chest pain who had a 12-lead electrocardiogram (ECG) performed

Measure #55 Electrocardiogram Performed for Syncope

Percentage of patients aged 60 years and older with an emergency department discharge diagnosis of syncope who had a 12-lead ECG performed

Measure #56 Vital Signs for Community-Acquired Bacterial Pneumonia

Percentage of patients aged 18 years and older with a diagnosis of community –acquired bacterial pneumonia with vital signs documented and reviewed

Measure #57 Assessment of Oxygen Saturation of Community-Acquired Bacterial Pneumonia

Percentage of patients aged 18 years and older with a diagnosis of community-acquired bacterial pneumonia with oxygen saturation documented and reviewed

Measure #58 Assessment of Mental Status for Community-Acquired Bacterial Pneumonia

Percentage of patients aged 18 years and older with a diagnosis of community-acquired bacterial pneumonia with mental status assessed

Measure #59 Empiric Antibiotic for Community-Acquired Bacterial Pneumonia

Percentage of patients aged 18 years and older with a diagnosis of community-acquired bacterial pneumonia with an appropriate empiric antibiotic prescribed

Measure #76 Prevention of Catheter-Related Bloodstream Infections (CRBSI) – Central Venous Catheter Insertion Protocol

Percentage of patients, regardless of age, who undergo central venous catheter (CVC) insertion for who CVC was inserted with all elements of maximal sterile barrier technique (cap AND mask AND sterile gown AND sterile gloves AND a large sterile sheet AND hand hygiene AND 2% chlorhexidine for cutaneous antisepsis followed).

Measure #91: Acute Otitis Externa (AOE): Topical Therapy

Percentage of patients aged 2 years and older with a diagnosis of AOE who were prescribed topical preparations

Measure #92: Acute Otitis Externa (AOE): Pain Assessment

Percentage of patient visits for those patients aged 2 years and older with a diagnosis of AOE with assessment for auricular or periauricular pain

Measure #93: Acute Otitis Externa (AOE): Systemic Antimicrobial Therapy – Avoidance of Inappropriate Use

Percentage of patients aged 2 years and older with a diagnosis of AOE who were not prescribed systemic antimicrobial therapy

Measure #252: Anticoagulation for Acute Pulmonary Embolus Patients

Anticoagulation ordered for patients who have been discharged from the emergency department (ED) with a diagnosis of acute pulmonary embolus. This measure is to be reported each time a patient has been discharged from the emergency department (i.e., transferred to another unit within the facility, transferred to another facility, or discharged to home) with a discharge diagnosis of acute pulmonary embolus during the reporting period.

Measure #253: Pregnancy Test for Female Abdominal Pain Patients

Percentage of female patients aged 14 to 50 who present to the emergency department (ED) with a chief complaint of abdominal pain for whom a pregnancy test is ordered. This measure is to be reported each time a female patient aged 14 to 50 presents to the emergency department with a chief complaint of abdominal pain. The patient should have documentation in the medical record of having a pregnancy test (urine or serum) ordered in the emergency department.

Measure #254: Ultrasound Determination of Pregnancy Location for Pregnant Patients with Abdominal Pain

Percentage of pregnant female patients aged 14 to 50 who present to the emergency department (ED) with a chief complaint of abdominal pain or vaginal bleeding who receive a trans-abdominal or trans-vaginal ultrasound to determine pregnancy location.

Measure #255: Rh Immunoglobulin (Rhogam) for Rh-Negative Pregnant Women at Risk of Fetal Blood Exposure

Percentage of Rh-negative pregnant women aged 14-50 years at risk of fetal blood exposure who receive Rh-Immunoglobulin (Rhogam) in the emergency department (ED). This measure is to be reported each time a pregnant patient presents to the emergency department with complaints including blunt abdominal trauma, vaginal bleeding, ectopic pregnancy, and threatened or spontaneous abortion. Patients who present to the emergency department with these complaints should have documentation in the medical record of receiving an order for Rh-Immunoglobulin (Rhogam).

5

EVALUATION AND MANAGEMENT (E&M) LEVELS

Each patient seen in the ED must pay for the services they receive. The bill that is generated from an ED visit depends on the level of care that is given. Simple medical cases that require less management and time will be billed for less than more complex cases. In order to be properly reimbursed for all services, physicians must properly document all cases. Unfortunately, charts do not always contain all necessary elements for reimbursement and are "down coded". This means that a hospital will not be properly reimbursed for the services rendered by the physician. The use of scribes has been shown to increase reimbursement for each chart due to charts being more complete. A scribe's primary responsibility is documentation so all details of the physician- patient encounter should be documented, and all charts must be complete and as detailed as possible. Charts are "coded" based on 5 E/M Levels. A chart is assigned level 1 for the simplest medical conditions, and a level 5 for the most complex medical cases. Keep in mind that in the ED patients are often assigned priority levels (1-5) based on their acuity level. These acuity levels are the opposite numbering as charting levels. For example, an acute MI would be assigned a level 1 priority and should always be a level 5 coded chart. An ankle injury may be assigned a level 3 or 4 priority and would be a level 3 coded chart. A simple suture removal would be a level 1 chart.

Coding levels require certain elements as follows:

Level 1: 1 element of the HPI and 1 element of the physical exam required. These patients may be seen in triage and leave immediately.

Example: suture removals or immunizations

Level 2: 1 element of the HPI, 1 element of the ROS, and 2 elements in the physical exam are required. These are considered "fast track" patients. They will be seen by a mid-level provider such as a PA or a NP if available.

Example: Localized rash such as poison ivy

Level 3: 1 element of the HPI, 1 element of the ROS, and 2 elements of the physical exam required. These patients will be discharged after receiving treatment.

Example: Wrist injury with possible fracture, Gastritis

Level 4: 4 elements of the HPI, 2 elements of the ROS, 1 element from PMH/SH/FH, and 5 elements from the physical exam required. These patients may or may not be admitted. They often require labs and one radiology study.

Example: Flank pain with dysuria, vaginal bleeding during pregnancy with abdominal cramping

Level 5: 4 elements of the HPI, 10 elements of the ROS, 2 elements from PMH/SH/FH, and 8 elements from the physical exam are required. Any patient that is likely to be admitted to the hospital should have a level 5 chart.

Example: Trauma, chest pain suspicious for cardiac etiology.

E/M Level	HPI	ROS	PMH / SH / FH	Physical Exam
Level 1	1	0	0	1
Level 2	1	1	0	2
Level 3	1	1	0	2
Level 4	4	2	1	5
Level 5	4	10	2	8

Additional elements of the chart also contribute to the reimbursement, which will be discussed further in the following sections.

6

AN OVERVIEW OF THE EMERGENCY DEPARTMENT

Understanding the emergency department will help you to optimize your role as a scribe and facilitate efficiency in the department. Each location will vary, and you will learn the specifics of your ED during your clinical training. The following includes general information and guidelines that will help you be a successful member of the emergency department.

Staff

The ED is composed of many different staff members, each with a unique role and responsibility. As a scribe, you are primarily interacting with the physician however, it is important that you understand the roles of others in the ED as you will be interacting with them from time to time.

Nurses

The have a multitude of responsibilities in the ED. They are assigned a few beds each, and maintain contact with their patients throughout their ED stay. There will often be a nurse who oversees the entire ED, known as the "charge nurse". It is important that you know who the charge nurse is. At times the charge nurse may ask you the status of your physician's patients and you must be able to communicate this information to him/her. The nurses may also ask you to relay messages to the physician if the physician is tied up elsewhere. Maintain a friendly, professional and respectful attitude when communicating with the nurses. If the physician asks you to relay a message to a nurse, always be respectful and keep in mind you are a messenger and not the one giving the instructions.

ED Techs

Techs are involved in much of the direct patient care including establishing IVs, drawing blood, and obtaining EKGs. They do not administer medication.

Radiology technicians

The individuals who perform XR, CT, US. They may come to the ED to clarify why a test is ordered, or specifically what the physician is looking for on a particular study.

Physician Assistant (PA)

See their own patients, can diagnose, treat and prescribe medication to patients. The PA will often work in the "fast track" area of the emergency department and see lower acuity cases; however, this varies by location.

Nurse Practitioner (NP)

A nurse with an advanced degree that will see patients on his/her own, under the supervision of the physician.

Registration Clerk

Checks patients into the ED, assigns patient number, verifies insurance information

ER Secretary

Answers the main ED phone, places pages, notifies of bed availability for admitted patients among many other responsibilities. This person will know all phone numbers of any department or person that you may need to call in the hospital. For example, if the ED physician is admitting a patient you may ask the secretary to page the admitting physician.

Work flow

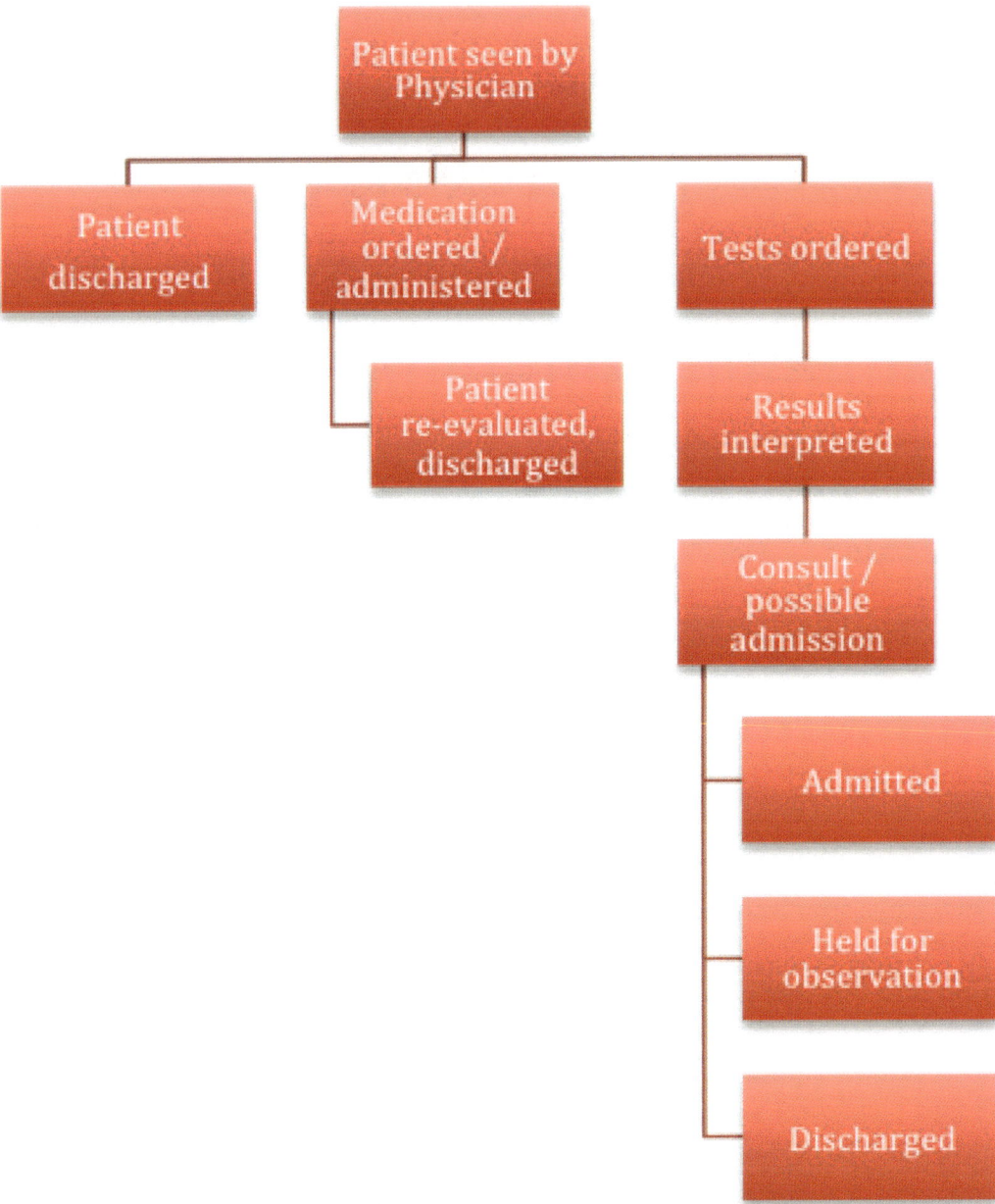

7

MEDICAL SCRIBE RESPONSIBILITIES

Documentation

As a medical scribe, you are not to be involved in direct patient care. Your role is strictly clerical and it is important to adhere to this rule. While in a patient's room, the physician may introduce you and may explain your role. You are to observe and document the interaction between the physician and patient. You are not to talk to the patient or the physician while in the patient's room unless the physician directly addresses you. If you have any questions regarding the information, you are to wait until you exit the room and ask the physician at this time. Never ask the patient your own questions. Do not hesitate to ask your physician questions in order to document the most accurate, detailed information possible. In addition, you should never provide the patient or family members with any information regarding test results or the medical plan. This is the physician's role, and strictly outside of your responsibilities.

The electronic medical record (EMR) is the computerized health record of each patient. It contains all of the patient's medical information within a given health system. At this point in time, EMRs are specific to locations, so health records from one facility will not be available within the EMR of another facility. Your main responsibility as a scribe is to create an ED physician note that will become a permanent part of the patient's health record in the EMR. The medical chart provides an account of all medical management and care the patient receives. It is a legal document that can be used in a court of law. In other words, should a medical case be the subject of a civil or criminal lawsuit, the EMR can be used as legal evidence. Therefore, accuracy is crucial in every record. If you ever identify a discrepancy within the chart, or are unsure of a detail ASK the physician for clarification. If a scribe is found to consistently make mistakes, this will likely lead to termination of the scribe. Remember, the chart is a part of the patient's permanent medical record and accuracy is essential.

As a scribe, be sure to adhere to the following guidelines:
- Always double check spelling for accuracy, especially when it comes to physician names and medications. Spelling and grammar errors are unacceptable.
- If you are unsure of a detail in the chart either from the patient's own account or the physician's remarks always be sure to ask the physician for clarification.

- The chart should always be readable by all members of the medical team. Therefore, you should limit use of abbreviations. If you do use abbreviations, only approved medical abbreviations are acceptable (refer to list in this manual). Never use any of your own abbreviations or abbreviations found in other resources. If you are unsure about using an abbreviation, it is best to not use it.

Other Duties

Pre-patient checklist
a.   Check the patient's room number to be sure the correct patient and chart are linked
b.   Turn off the television to eliminate all distractions in the room

Post-patient checklist
a.   As patient studies are available, you should alert the physician. At this time you may also prompt the physician for any update he or she would like included in the chart, and inquire about a possible plan for the patient.
b.   Verify and record what tests are being ordered (labs and radiology).
c.   Check off tests as the results become available.
d.   Record any EKG, pulse-ox, or rhythm strip information. Ask physician for this information.

Keeping track of tests
a.   Alert the physician of any abnormal lab values. If available, you should look in the patient's records to see if prior lab studies are available for comparison. You should present this information to the physician along with new lab values, especially any significantly changed values.

For example, if a patient's hemoglobin level is 9 g/dL, you should look for any previous hemoglobin levels. If you see a value from 6 months prior that was 12 g/dL and another value a year before of 11.7 g/dL you would know that this value of 9 g/dL is lower than the patient's typical hemoglobin level. You could alert the physician by saying, "Mr. X's hemoglobin is a 9. I looked in his prior studies and found that he typically runs around 12." This gives the physician information about the current lab value in the context of the patient's medical history.

b. Notifying physician when any radiology test is available. If applicable pull up the images for the physician to review.

c. Notifying physician when all tests are complete

d. Do not import laboratory or radiology studies into the chart until the physician has seen them.

e. If a particular study is taking longer than usual to obtain, call the lab on your own to inquire about the results or expected time to results. At times lab may be delayed if a sample is hemolyzed, or if the wrong colored tube was sent for a particular test. In the event that this has occurred you may politely inform the nurse or physician so that the proper sample may be sent.

f. If a patient ever asks for directions to the restroom, be sure they have provided any necessary urine samples before directing him or her. If they have not provided a sample, you may ask them to do so and then inform a nurse or tech. Never handle a urine sample from a patient.

Keeping physician on track

a. As patient studies are available, you should alert the physician. At this time you may also prompt the physician for any update he or she would like included in the chart, and inquire about a possible plan for the patient.

b. Throughout the patient's stay you should know if he or she is likely to be discharged or admitted. As results are completed, you should prompt the physician to "dispo" the patient and either work on getting the patient admitted or discharge the patient.

c. If a patient is being admitted, you should be sure that all admission criteria are properly documented. More details regarding this is provided in the appendix.

d. You are overseeing all of the physician's patients and their progress in the ED. Part of your role as a scribe is to ensure a patient's care is not being delayed for any reason. Therefore, take any necessary steps to facilitate efficiency in the ED.

Writing discharge instructions
a. If a patient is discharged from the emergency room, they will be given discharge instructions. Your role as a scribe includes putting together these instructions, as well as follow up instructions per the physician's request.

Looking up records
a. It is sometimes helpful to view records from a patient's recent ED visit or hospitalization. For example, if a patient is seen in the ED multiple times for the same complaint, looking at these records may provide the physician with insight into types of treatment that may work for the patient. If possible, you should scan the patient's chart for this type of information, and present any relevant information to the physician.
b. It is also useful to see recent relevant medical tests that a patient may have had. For example, if a patient comes in with chest pain it would be helpful to know if they had any prior cardiac evaluations such as a stress test, echo, or cardiac cath. If these records exist you should inform your physician of the test and any pertinent results.
c. Only look up records that are pertinent to the visit at hand. For example, if a patient presents to the ED for abdominal pain, do not open up a note describing their knee replacement surgery. This would be a violation of HIPPA.

8

THE MEDICAL CHART: SOAP NOTES

SUBJECTIVE (S)

The subjective part of the chart is any information provided by the patient or anyone else giving information about the patient (i.e. family members, friends, EMS, home health worker). This portion of the chart includes the patient's account of why they are presenting to the emergency room as well as their medical history.

1. History of Presenting Illness (HPI)

The HPI is the account of why a patient is presenting to the emergency department from his or her own perspective. At times, the patient's story will be long and may contain irrelevant facts. The physician will ask the patient questions to help organize the story, which will help direct the type of care the patient will receive. It is your responsibility to listen carefully to this interaction and write a coherent medical history. There are important details to include in the HPI that will not only help in coding the chart, but also help other medical personnel understand the patient's story in medical terms. The chief complain is the main reason the person is presenting to the ED, for example, abdominal pain or chest pain. The rest of the HPI describes the events that led the patient to come to the ED.

Important details to include are:

- Location: where is the pain?

- Radiation: Does the pain go anywhere else?

- Onset: When did the pain begin? Was it gradual or sudden?

- Duration: How long does the pain last? Seconds/minutes/ hours

- Course: Has the pain been improving/constant/worsening?

- Severity: Rate the pain on a scale of 1-10, is it mild/moderate/severe?

- Quality: Describe the pain. i.e. sharp/dull/achy/ burning/pressure/ throbbing

- Context: What causes the pain to come on? i.e. movement/ exertion/ palpation

- Modifying factors: Does anything make the pain better or worse?

- Associated symptoms: Is the pain associated with any other symptoms? i.e. nausea, vomiting, sweats, headache, chills

In a level 5 chart, 4 of these elements must be included in the HPI.

The following is an example HPI for a patient presenting with chest pain:

45 y/o otherwise healthy male presents to the ED via EMS c/o substernal chest pain (location) for the past 2 days (onset). The pt states that the pain has been fluctuating in intensity (course) from a 3/10 at minimum to a 9/10 at maximum (severity) and is associated with exertion (context). He describes the pain as "pressure" (quality) and denies any radiation. He states the pain is exacerbated by exertion such as climbing stairs (modifying factor) and is relieved by ASA (modifying factor). The pt reports some associated dyspnea and diaphoresis (associated symptoms). Denies nausea, vomiting, abdominal discomfort, chills, fever. He was given ASA by EMS just prior to arrival. He is currently asymptomatic. Family history of CAD with father MI in the 50s. Pt is a current 1ppd smoker.

2. Review of Systems (ROS)

This is a comprehensive list of the body's systems. The doctor will ask the patient if they have had any other recent complaints that may or may not be related to the patient's chief complaint. This list should be documented in the "ROS" section. Any specific complaint that the patient identifies or denies should be explicitly indicated. Any symptom that pertains to the CC should be documented in the HPI in addition to the ROS.

There are 14 systems and symptoms will be grouped accordingly due to the following:

- Allergy/immunology: ex: seasonal allergies, swollen lymph nodes

- Cardiovascular: ex: chest pain, diaphoresis, palpitations, tachycardia, syncope

- Constitutional: ex: fever, chills, decreased appetite, generalized weakness, fatigue

- HENT: ex: ear ache, sore throat, rhinorrhea

- Eye: ex: photophobia, diplopia, blurred vision

- Endocrine: ex: excessive urination (polyuria), hypoglycemia, hyperglycemia

- Gastrointestinal: ex: Abdominal pain, nausea, vomiting, diarrhea, constipation

- Genitourinary: ex: vaginal bleeding, testicular pain, dysuria, hematuria

- Hematologic/Lymphatic: ex: bruising tendency, bleeding tendency

- Integumentary (skin): ex: rash, dryness

- Musculoskletal: ex: pain, swelling, decreased ROM

- Neurologic: ex: altered coordination, altered speech, dizziness, headache

- Psychiatric: ex: depression, insomnia, suicidal ideation

- Respiratory: ex: cough, wheezing, sputum production

The preceding list includes the systems and examples of symptoms from each. If the physician specifically asks about a complaint, you should document this. For example, if the physician asks a patient if he or she has had a recent cough and the patient says no, the scribe would document in the respiratory section "Patient denies recent cough." If a patient for some reason is unable to answer the physician's questions, the scribe should document, "review of systems unable to be obtained due to the patient's clinical status". If the patient regains consciousness after the physician's initial evaluation, the ROS remains "unable to be obtained." The scribe should document at what time the patient regains consciousness and any changes of the ROS or PE.

In a level 5 chart, 10/14 systems must be reviewed.

3.   **Additional History**

- Past Medical History: What are the patient's previous medical conditions? i.e. HTN, CAD, DM, anxiety, COPD

In our sample patient, he was described as "otherwise healthy" which is another way of saying he has no contributory medical history to his case. In this case he did not have any underlying medical conditions.

- Surgical History: What are the patient's prior surgeries? i.e. cardiac stents, appendectomy, hip replacement

In our sample patient he may have has a h/o a wrist fracture repair. We would document this in the surgical history section, but since it is not cardiac related it would not be included in the HPI.

- Social History: Does the patient smoke or drink? Is the patient employed? Who does the patient live with?

We mentioned that the sample patient was a 1 ppd (pack per day) smoker.

- Family History: Does the patient have any close relatives (i.e. parents, siblings, grandparents) with medical conditions? It is especially important to note if the patient has a family member with a condition related to the chief complaint.

In our patient we mentioned his family h/o CAD and a father with an MI in his 50s. This family history would be considered "contributory" to the patient's current problem and was thus commented on in his HPI in addition to this section.

- Allergies : Does the patient have any known drug allergies? It is especially important to take note of any latex, medication, or contrast dye allergy as these are commonly used in the ED.

In this case he did not therefore we would document NKA (no known allergies)

- Medications: What daily medications does the patient currently take?

This patient does not take daily medications. If a patient does take medications it is important to document the medications and the dosages.

- Immunizations: Are the patient's immunizations up to date? This is especially important for patients at risk for tetanus such as lacerations or animal bites.

This patient's immunizations are UTD (up to date).

- LMP: This section is only for female patients. You would document the status of the patient's menses i.e. the LMP, if the patient is menopausal or if the patient has had a hysterectomy.

The past history can give the physician insight into types of medical conditions the patient may be at risk for. It can also be helpful in directing a differential diagnosis. For example, if a patient with abdominal pain has a history of an appendectomy, the physician can exclude appendicitis as a possible etiology of the abdominal pain.

In a level 5 chart, at least 2 past history elements must be documented. However, it is good practice to always document as much information as possible in this section to provide the most complete medical picture.

OBJECTIVE (O)

This portion of the chart consists of objective, unbiased, findings. In includes the physical examination, vital signs, measurements, diagnostic test results, and any procedures.

1. **Physical Exam**

The physical exam is a head to toe examination of the patient performed by the physician. Findings are organized in the chart by organ system. A physician may have a standard "normal" physical exam, which you can use as a template. They will then note pertinent positives or negatives that they want included in the chart. Depending on the physician, he or she will either call out exam findings in the room for you to enter into the chart, or will discuss findings with you immediately after leaving the room. It is important that you pay attention during the exam to be sure everything the physician examines is documented, and that items that were not examined are not included. For example, if the physician's template includes "normal bowel sounds", but the physician did not listen to the patient's bowel sounds, you should take this out of the exam. The template is there to make you and your physician's job easier, but it is your responsibility as the scribe to be sure the exam documentation is accurate for each case.

The major body systems to listen for are:

- Constitutional

- Eyes

- Head

- Ears, Nose, Throat

- Cardiovascular

- Respiratory

- Gastrointestinal

- Genitourinary

- Musculoskeletal

- Chest wall

- Back

- Skin

- Neurologic

- Psychiatric

- Hematology, Lymphatic, Immunology

There are times where a patient may come in with a very specific complaint (ex: arm pain and swelling after falling onto an outstretched arm). In this case, the doctor will likely perform a focused exam that revolves around that arm, and will not include other systems.

Example examination for our sample patient:

- Constitutional: NAD, alert, well-appearing

- Eyes: Normal conjunctiva, PERRLA, EOMI

- Head: Normocephalic, atraumatic

- Ears, Nose, Throat: TM clear bilaterally, mucus membranes moist

- Cardiovascular: RRR, brisk capillary refill, no edema

- Respiratory: Lungs CTA, no respiratory distress, breath sounds equal

- Gastrointestinal: abdomen is soft, non-tender, non-distended

- Musculoskeletal: no swelling, no deformity

- Chest wall: chest pain is not reproduced by palpation of the chest wall

- Skin: warm, dry, normal for ethnicity

- Neurologic: CN II-XII grossly intact, no focal neurologic deficits, A&Ox3

- Psychiatric: cooperative, appropriate mood and affect

- Hematology, Lymphatic, Immunology: no lymphadenopathy

In a level 5 chart, at least 8 items must be documented in the physical exam.

2. **Vital Signs and Measurements**

Any vital signs including heart rate, blood pressure, pulse-ox, and temperature should be included in the chart. This may be obtained from the nurse's notes or from observation while in the examination room. If the doctor orders additional measurements such as orthostatic vital signs, these should be included in the chart. If a patient is on a cardiac monitor, you should document this as well.

Vital Signs:

- Blood pressure (BP)
    - Normal range: Approximately 100-130 systolic, 65-85 diastolic
    - Hypotensive: less than 100 systolic, less than 60 diastolic
    - Hypertensive: greater than 140 systolic, greater than 90 diastolic
    - These are just general ranges that vary depending on age, health status, medication, and environment. For example, the stress of being in an emergency department may cause a person's BP to increase slightly.
- Temperature: Approximately 98.6F is considered "normal".
    - An adult is considered febrile with a temperature above 101F (oral) and a child is considered febrile with a temperature above 100F (rectal).
- Respiratory rate (RR): In adults, normal RR is 12-18 breaths per minute.
    - Increased respiratory rate is called "tachypnea."
    - Children normally have a higher RR than adults which varies depending on age.
- Pulse-ox (oxygen saturation level): Normal values 95-100%. Important to note if this is while the patient is on room air (RA), or on oxygen (indicate how much oxygen patient is on).
    - Less than 90% is considered hypoxia, saturation levels in the low 90s are borderline hypoxia and should be increased.
    - Oxygen saturation levels vary in patients with lung diseases such as lung cancer or COPD (are usually lower than normal range).
- Heart Rate (HR)/ Pulse: Normal range in adults is 60-100 beats per minute (bpm)
    - Tachycardia: greater than 100 bpm
    - Bradycardia: less than 60 bpm
    - Athletes typically have lower resting heart rates than the average person
    - Children have higher HR than adults

3. Diagnostic studies

Any laboratory studies, urinalysis, EKG, or radiology tests should be included in the chart. Part of your role as a scribe is to keep track of tests ordered and to alert the physician as tests are complete. If a particular laboratory value or radiology test is taking longer than usual and is delaying the patient's care in the ED you should take any possible measures to obtain the result.

Example diagnostic studies for our patient:

EKG: NSR at 76bpm, no ST segment changes, no T wave abnormalities, unchanged from prior EKG 4/11/11

CXR: NADP

Labs: Cardiac enzymes, BMP, CBC: WNL

4. Medical Decision Making (MDM)

In this section of the chart the physician's decision-making process is explained. It usually begins with the differential diagnosis based on the history and examination. It then explains any tests ordered and the results of such tests. It includes treatments administered in the ED. It may also include additional information about the physician's decision making, including reasons for excluding certain diagnoses and plans for future management. The MDM is also an area to document any necessary CMS core measures, or admission criteria.

In this section of the chart, the physician's decision-making process is explained. It will be structured differently depending on the physician. Usually it begins with the differential diagnosis based on the history and examination. It then explains any tests ordered and the results of such tests. It includes treatments administered in the ED.
It may also include additional information about the physician's decision making, including reasons for excluding certain diagnoses and plans for future management. The MDM is also an area to document any necessary CMS core measures, or admission criteria.

In simple cases, you can write the MDM based on what the physician discusses with the patient in the room. Other cases will be more complex. In these situations you should document the main elements such as the DDx, labs, and medication given. You should then consult with the physician about anything else he or she would like documented. The more experience you have working, the better you will become at anticipating what to include in the MDM. In all cases you should listen carefully to the physician's discussion with the patient. This should give you most of the information that is important to include in the MDM.

Example MDM for this patient:

45 y/o male with non-specific chest pain. Pt was given ASA by EMS. DDx included angina, non-specific chest pain, MI, CAD, PE, MSK chest pain. Pt has some risk factors for ACS including family history and h/o smoking. Will obtain EKG, basic labs including cardiac markers, and CXR. If these studies are negative I recommend that the pt stay overnight in observation for a stress test in the morning.

CXR, cardiac enzymes and EKG all WNL. Pt has remained CP free throughout ED stay. I discussed the plan with pt along with smoking cessation. He understands and agrees to stay overnight in the cardiac observation unit for a stress test in the morning.

5.   Differential Diagnoses

A differential diagnosis is any explanation that the doctor has for the patient's symptoms that he or she will rule out by the various tests they ordered. The differential will either be dictated to you as its own separate section or be included in the medical decision making, depending on the physician's preference of how they would like to organize their chart.

ASSESSMENT/PLAN (AP)

1.   Diagnosis

Always be sure to put a diagnosis in the chart. This is important both for billing purposes and for admitting patients. If the physician does not tell you a diagnosis it is your responsibility to ask the physician for one. Never leave this portion of the note blank.

For this sample patient, the diagnosis would be: non-specific chest pain.

2.   Disposition

This is the ultimate plan for the patient. Will the patient be discharged, transferred to the care of the next attending physician, or admitted?
This is also where discharge and follow up instructions should be imported for any patient being discharged. Unless the physician states otherwise, you will be responsible for completing the discharge instructions and any necessary follow up information.

The sample patient: Patient will be admitted to the chest pain observation unit overnight for a stress test in the morning. If stress test is negative he is stable for discharge and is instructed to follow up with his PCP within the next week.

3.   Calls/ Consults

If the physician consults with any specialists or discusses the case with anyone, it should be documented here. Examples may include social workers, the patient's PCP, a specialist, or the admitting physician. In any consult document the time of the consultation, the person the consult was with, and any pertinent information obtained.

4.   Re-evaluation

Often times the physician will re-evaluate a patient during their hospital stay to assess whether or not they are improving with treatment. Any time the physician has contact with the patient it may be considered a re-evaluation. For any re-evaluation, document the time and any changes in the patient's condition.

Example re-evaluation:

Time: 1430
Course: The patient remains stable and in NAD. Vital signs are stable. Awaiting results of chest CT. If   negative, anticipate discharge.

5.   Other Charting Elements

Procedure Notes: Any procedures performed in the ED need to be documented in a separate section of the chart. A general procedure note should include the following elements:

- Time out/ consent: Who is the patient, what is the procedure, who consented (patient/ guardian/ parent), was it a written or verbal consent?

- Indication: Why is the procedure being performed?

- Preparation: Was there a prep? i.e. sterile field, cleansed with betadine/ chlorhexidine

- Medication: Were any medications used during the procedure?

- Technique: How was the procedure performed? i.e. Which part of the body the procedure was performed? What gauge needle used in a laceration repair, what type of sutures, how many sutures?

- Time: How long did the procedure take?

- Outcome: How did the patient tolerate the procedure? Was it successful? (i.e. was the dislocation re-located?

- Performed by: Who performed the procedure? Sometimes the physician will have a resident or medical perform a procedure to obtain experience. In this case you should document that a resident performed the procedure.

Common Procedures performed in the ED:

- I&D: Stands for Incision & Drainage; it is a procedure. Procedure to release pus/buildup under the skin caused by an abscess.

- Conscious sedation: Accompanies another procedure, but must be documented separately. It is done when a patient needs to be temporarily sedated while another procedure is being performed.

- Fracture/dislocation reduction: Performed to re-align a displaced fracture or relocate a dislocated joint.

- Laceration repair: Suture or glue repair of a laceration

- Endotracheal Intubation: Procedure performed to protect the airway in a patient in severe respiratory distress or who for some reason cannot breath on his or her own. A tube is placed down the patient's throat and attached to a ventilator.

- Central Line Placement: A tube placed directly into a vein to establish IV access. This procedure is done in order to administer certain medications or to establish long term IV access.

- Lumbar puncture (LP): A sample of cerebrospinal fluid is taken from the patient. It is performed in a sterile environment by inserting a needle between the patient's vertebral discs. CSF is then analyzed for the possibility of meningitis, or occult blood not seen on a CT in the event of a cerebral hemorrhage. This may also be done to relieve intracranial pressure.

6. **Critical Care Notes**

For patients with high acuity, complex cases it may be necessary for the physician to spend more time on the case than with a "typical" case. In these situations, it is possible for the physician to bill for "critical care time" based on the services and time spent. Critical care time can be billed for more RVUs than typical care time. The first increment of critical care is 30-74 minutes and each additional 30 minutes is billed in increments. Since critical care time receives additional reimbursement, it has certain elements that must be met in order to meet the billing requirements.

Components that must be met in order to bill for critical care:
1. There is evidence of a critical illness in which 1 or more vital organ system is in danger of deterioration, which is life threatening for the patient.
2. The physician is directly involved in interventions
3. At least 30 minutes is involved in the patient's care including:
    a. Direct bedside care
    b. Documentation time (in the case of a scribe, time spent discussing the case with the scribe will count towards this)
    c. Discussion with other medical staff
    d. Time spent reviewing labs/ radiology/ old records
    e. Time spent discussing the case with family members/ caretakers if the patient is unable to communicate

It is important to note that the time spent on the previous items does not need to be in succession, as the physician will likely also be caring for other patients in the department. Therefore, the time is considered an approximation. In critical care patients it is also important to include frequent re-evaluations of the patient in order to properly document the time spent caring for the patient. In addition, any discussion with other medical personnel should be documented.

The following procedures can be billed separately from critical care, and therefore cannot be included in the critical care time:

- Endotracheal intubation
- Central line placement

When recording critical care, be sure to document all documents reviewed, all tests ordered and their interpretations, all consults, and any other element of care that was performed. Since critical care receives higher reimbursements these notes are more likely to be audited, therefore accuracy is imperative.

9

BASIC ANATOMY

A. Head

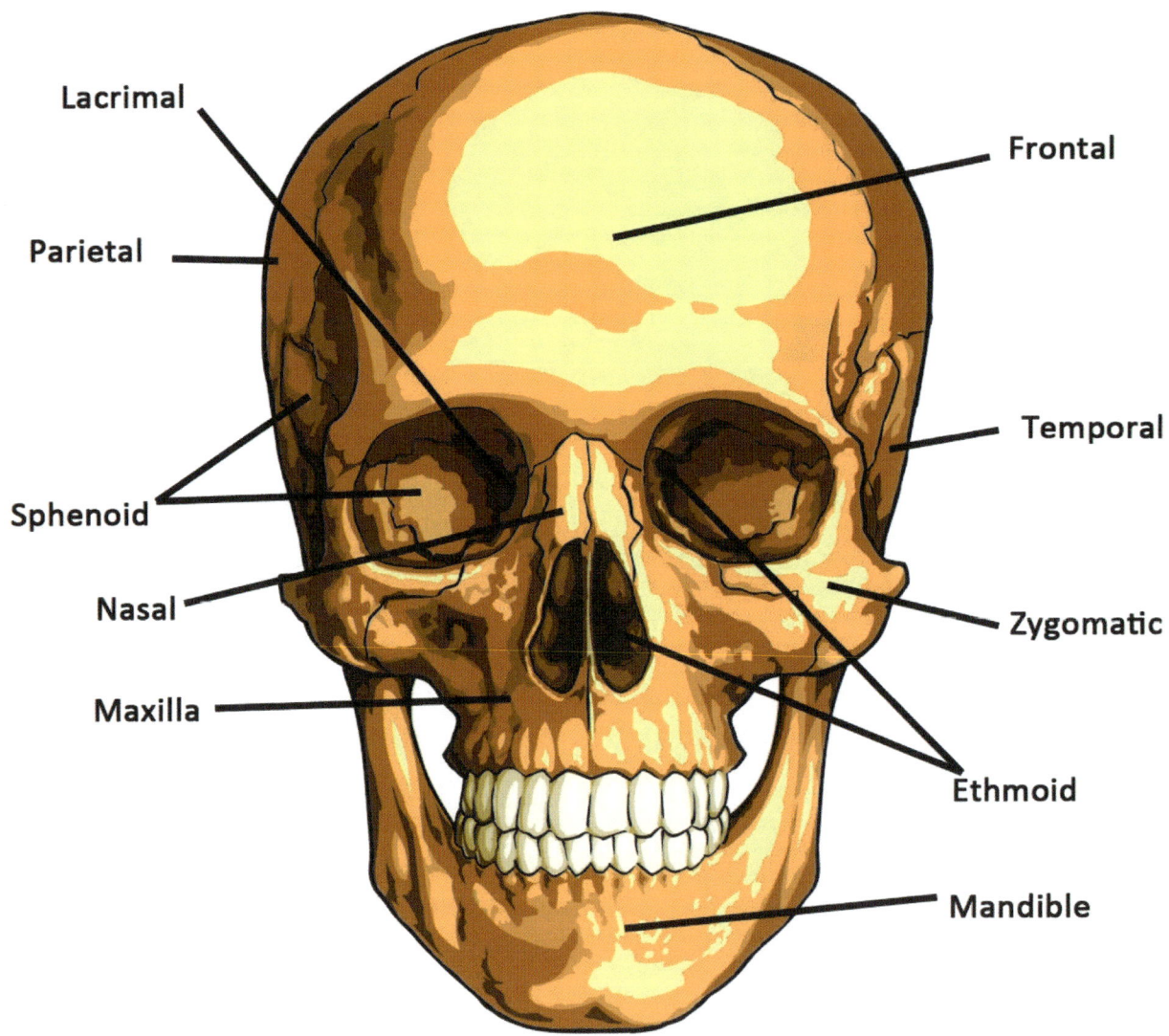

Lacrimal

Frontal

Parietal

Temporal

Sphenoid

Nasal

Zygomatic

Maxilla

Ethmoid

Mandible

B. Neck / Back

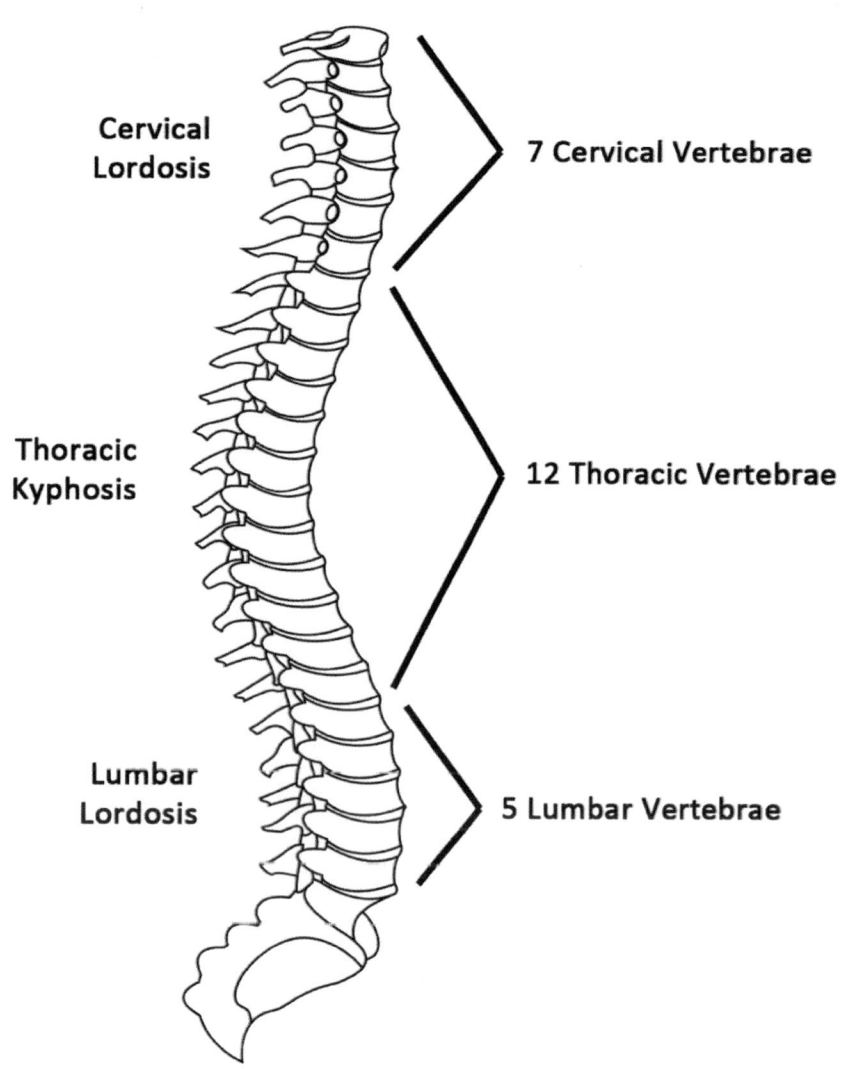

Cervical
Lordosis

7 Cervical Vertebrae

Thoracic
Kyphosis

12 Thoracic Vertebrae

Lumbar
Lordosis

5 Lumbar Vertebrae

C. Skeletal System

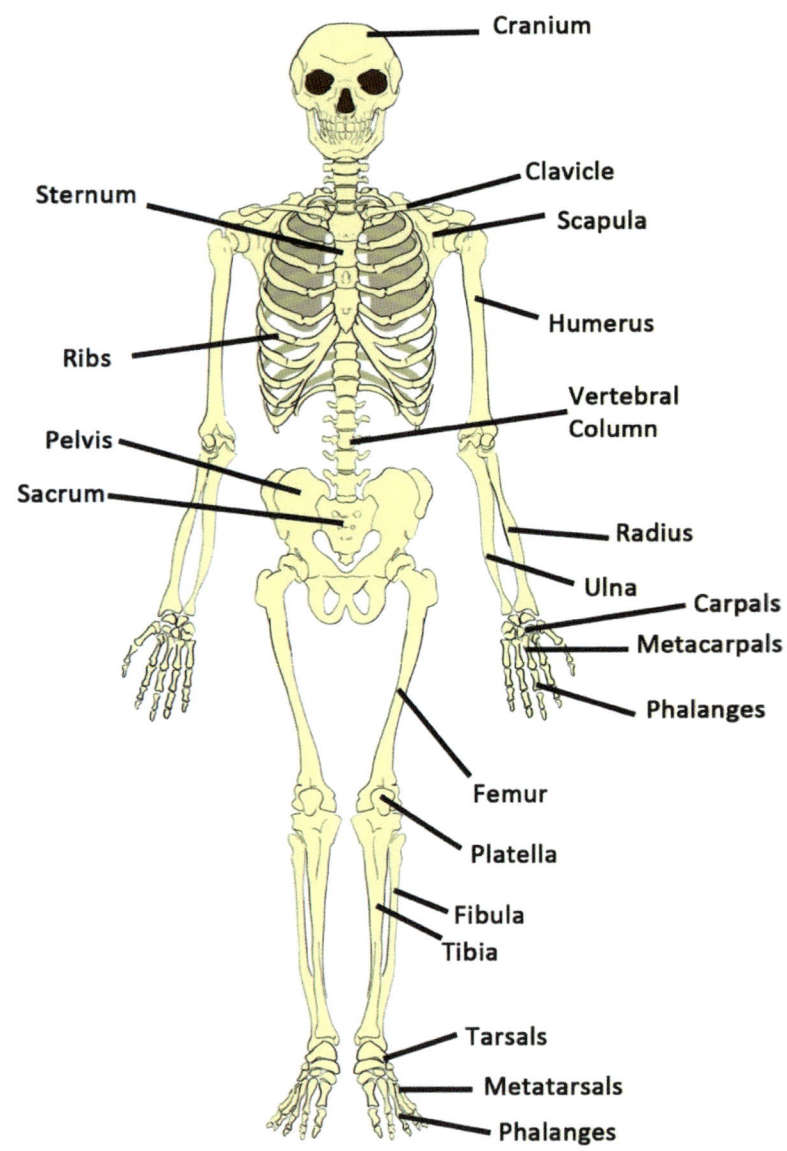

Cranium

Clavicle

Sternum

Scapula

Humerus

Ribs

Vertebral Column

Pelvis

Sacrum

Radius

Ulna

Carpals

Metacarpals

Phalanges

Femur

Platella

Fibula

Tibia

Tarsals

Metatarsals

Phalanges

D. Digestive System

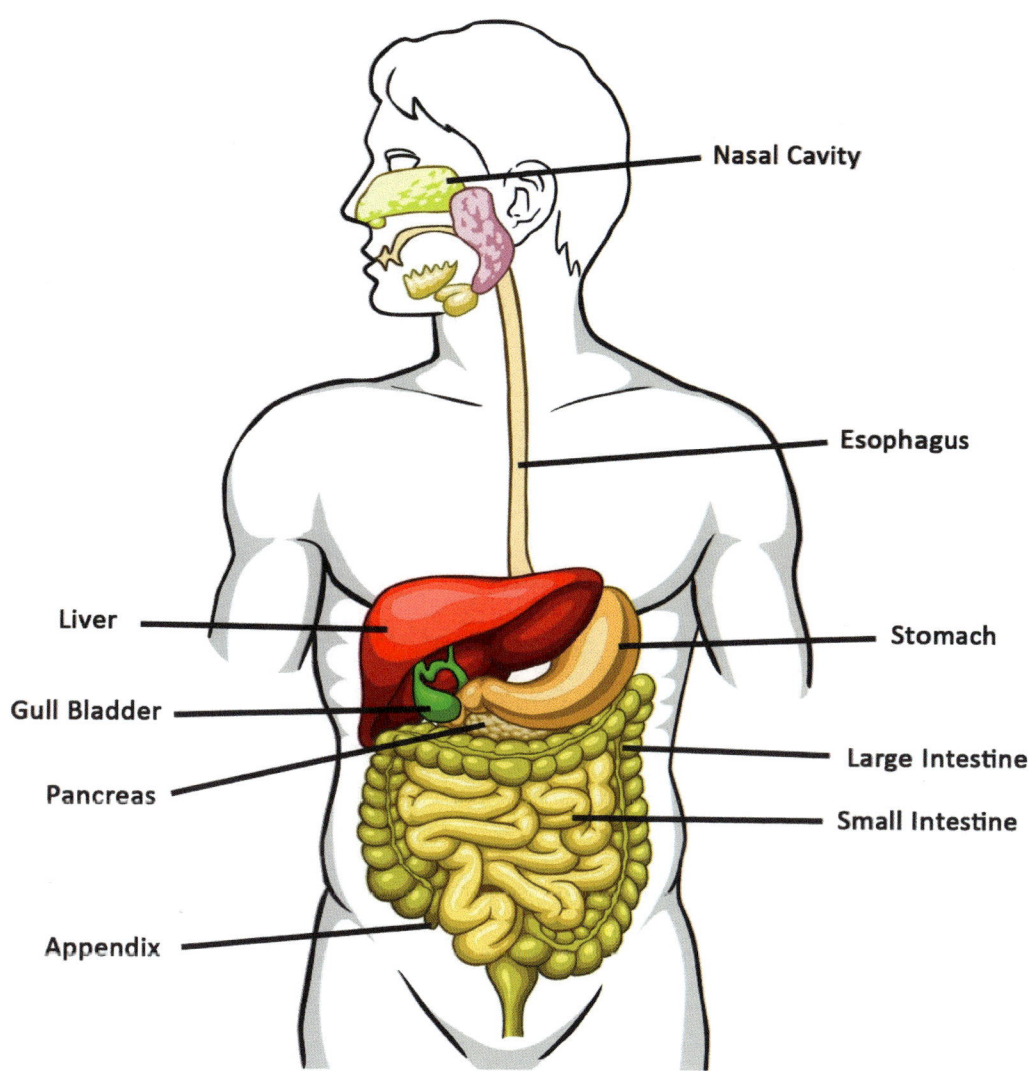

Nasal Cavity

Esophagus

Liver

Stomach

Gull Bladder

Pancreas

Large Intestine

Small Intestine

Appendix

E. Lungs

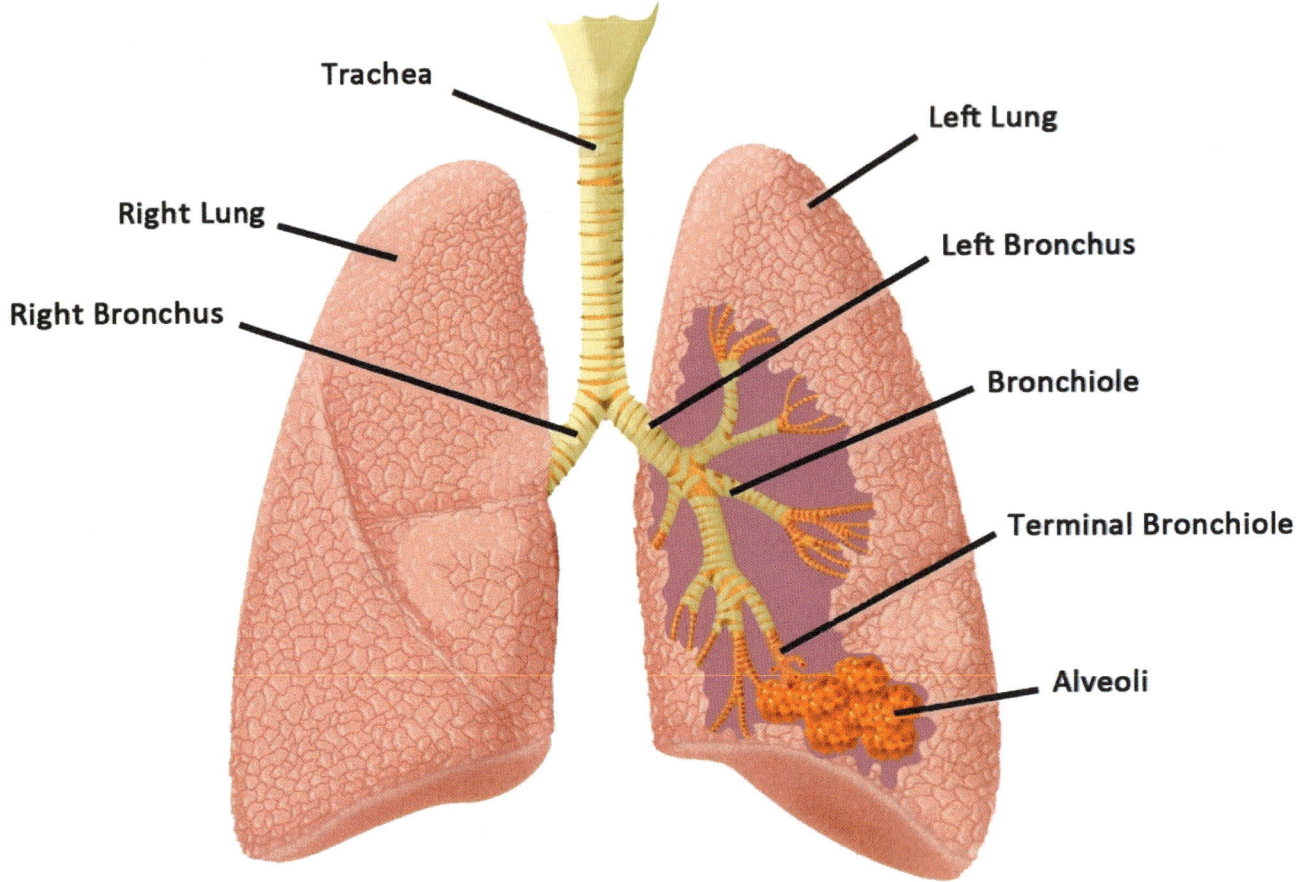

Trachea

Left Lung

Right Lung

Left Bronchus

Right Bronchus

Bronchiole

Terminal Bronchiole

Alveoli

F. Heart

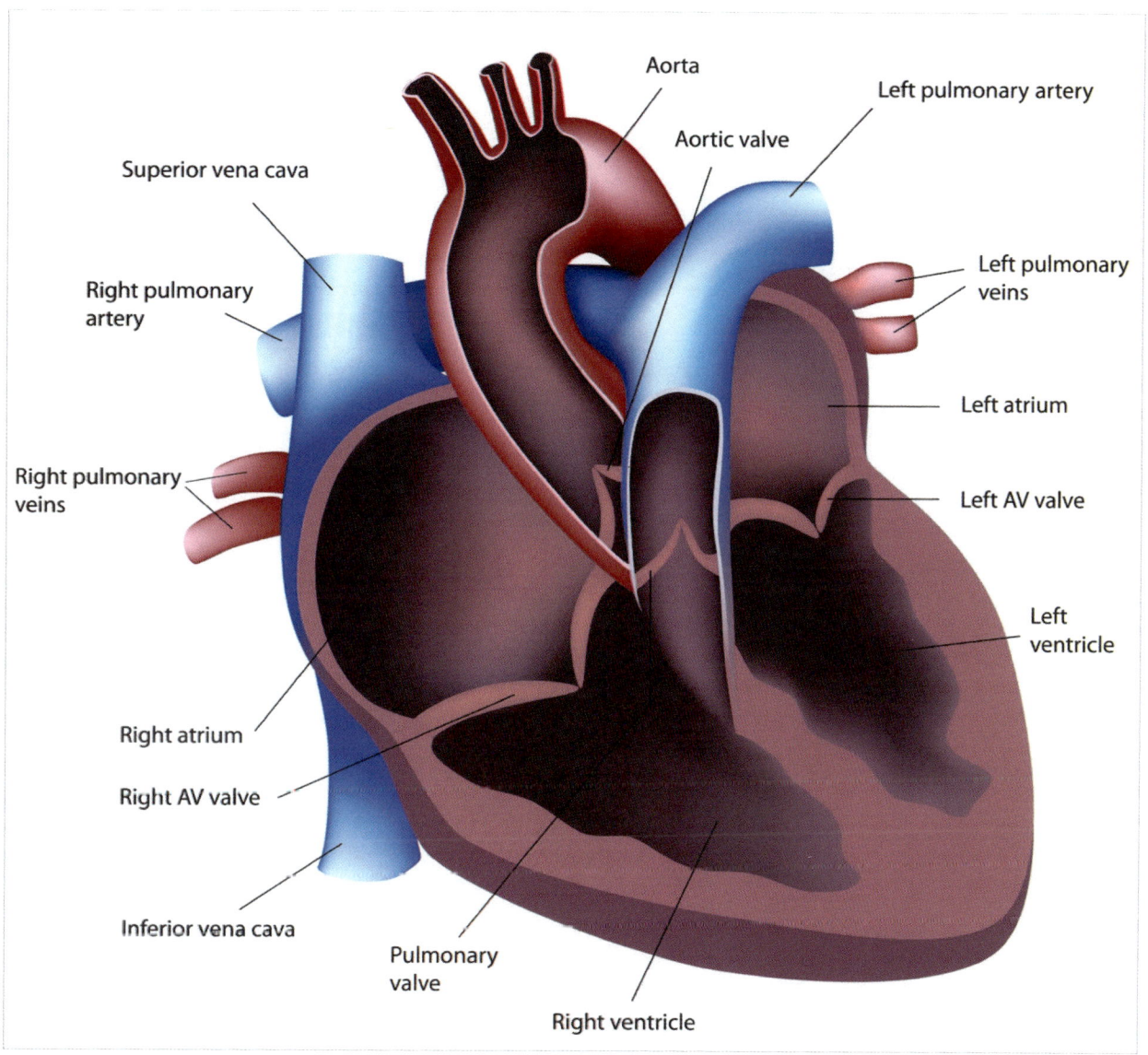

Aorta

Aortic valve

Left pulmonary artery

Superior vena cava

Left pulmonary veins

Right pulmonary artery

Left atrium

Right pulmonary veins

Left AV valve

Right atrium

Left ventricle

Right AV valve

Inferior vena cava

Pulmonary valve

Right ventricle

G. Muscular System (Front)

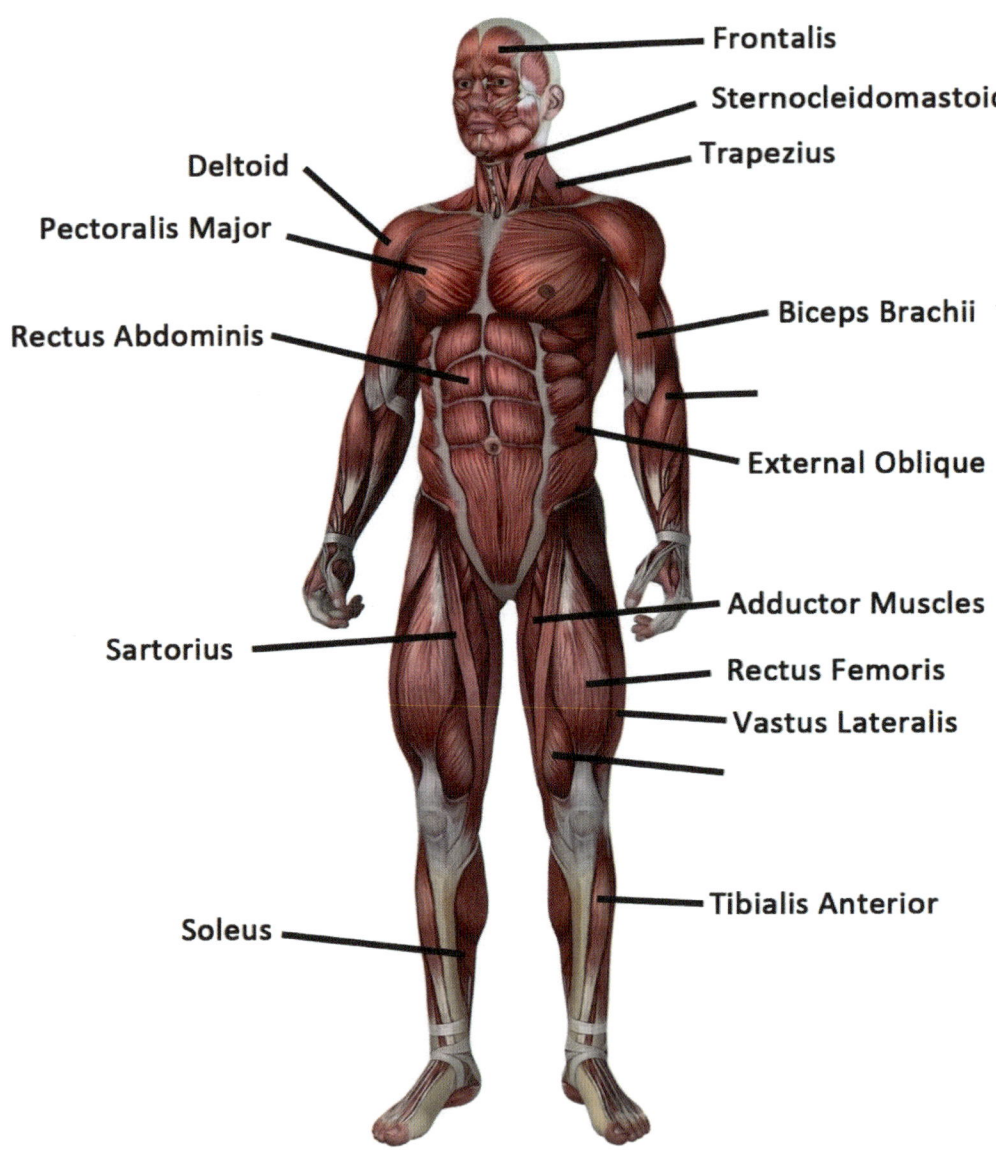

Frontalis

Sternocleidomastoid

Trapezius

Deltoid

Pectoralis Major

Biceps Brachii

Rectus Abdominis

External Oblique

Adductor Muscles

Sartorius

Rectus Femoris

Vastus Lateralis

Tibialis Anterior

Soleus

H. Muscular System (Back)

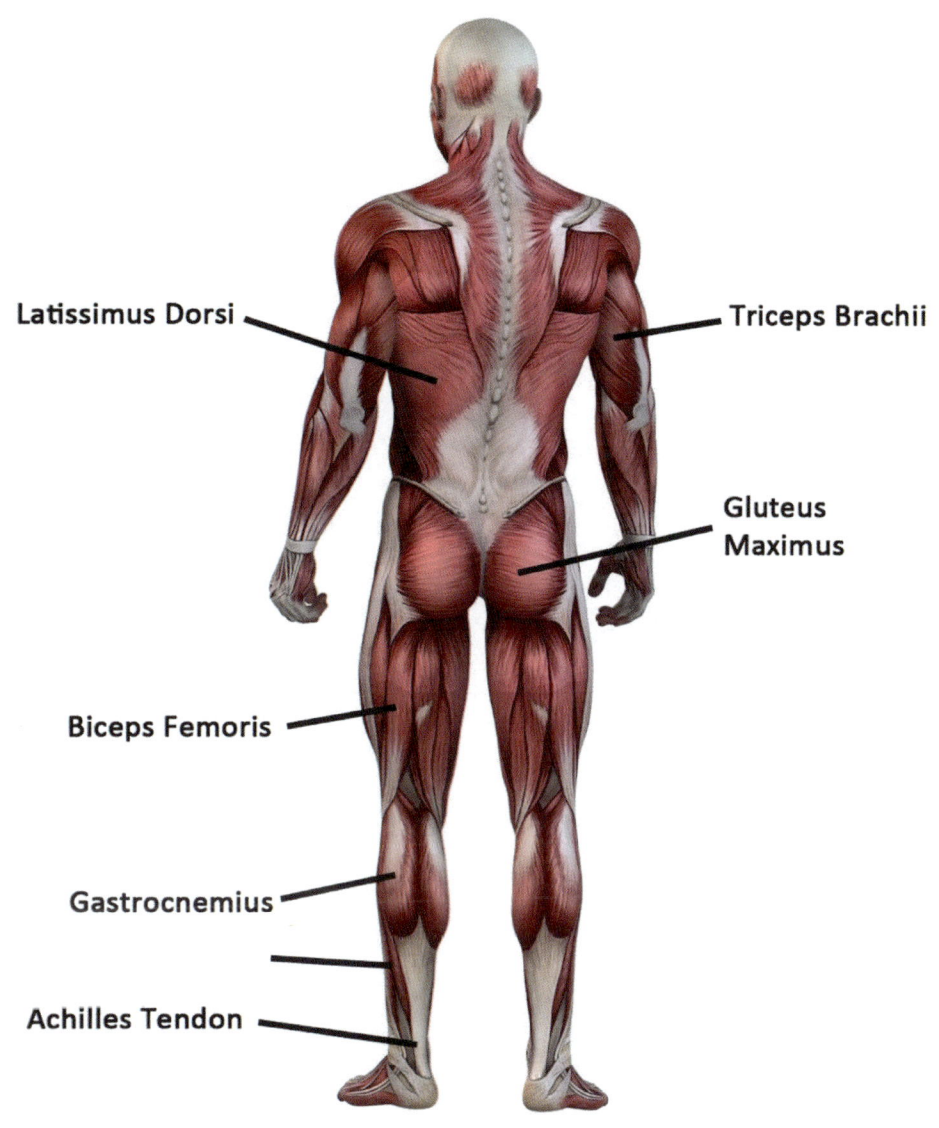

Latissimus Dorsi

Triceps Brachii

Gluteus Maximus

Biceps Femoris

Gastrocnemius

Achilles Tendon

I. Male Reproductive System

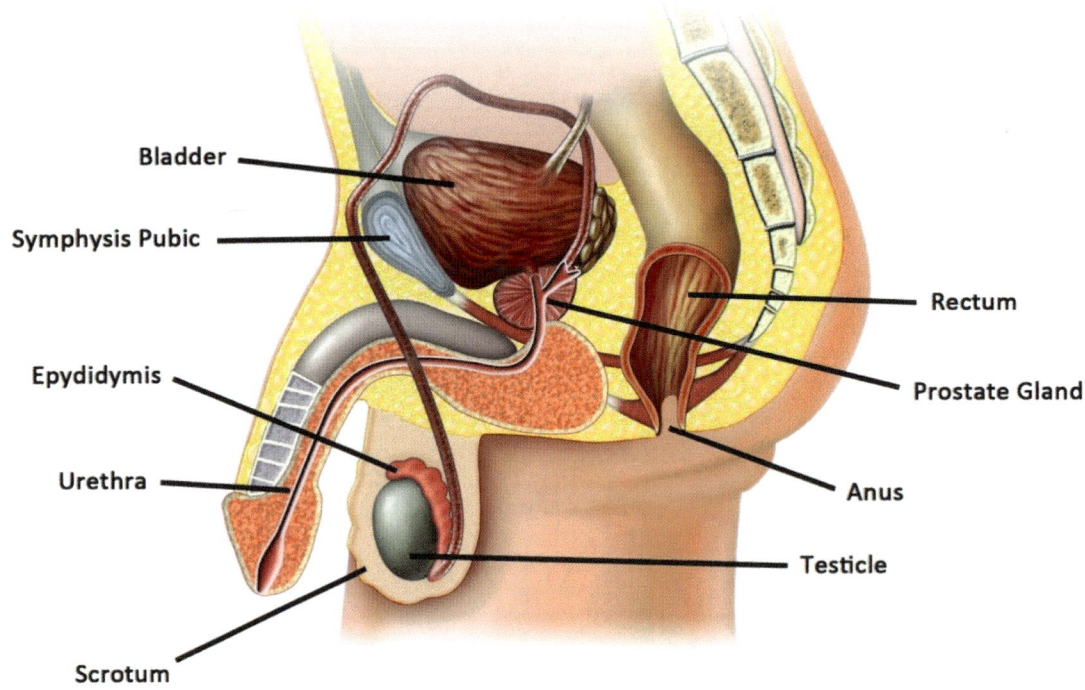

Bladder

Symphysis Pubic

Epydidymis

Urethra

Scrotum

Rectum

Prostate Gland

Anus

Testicle

J. Female Reproductive System

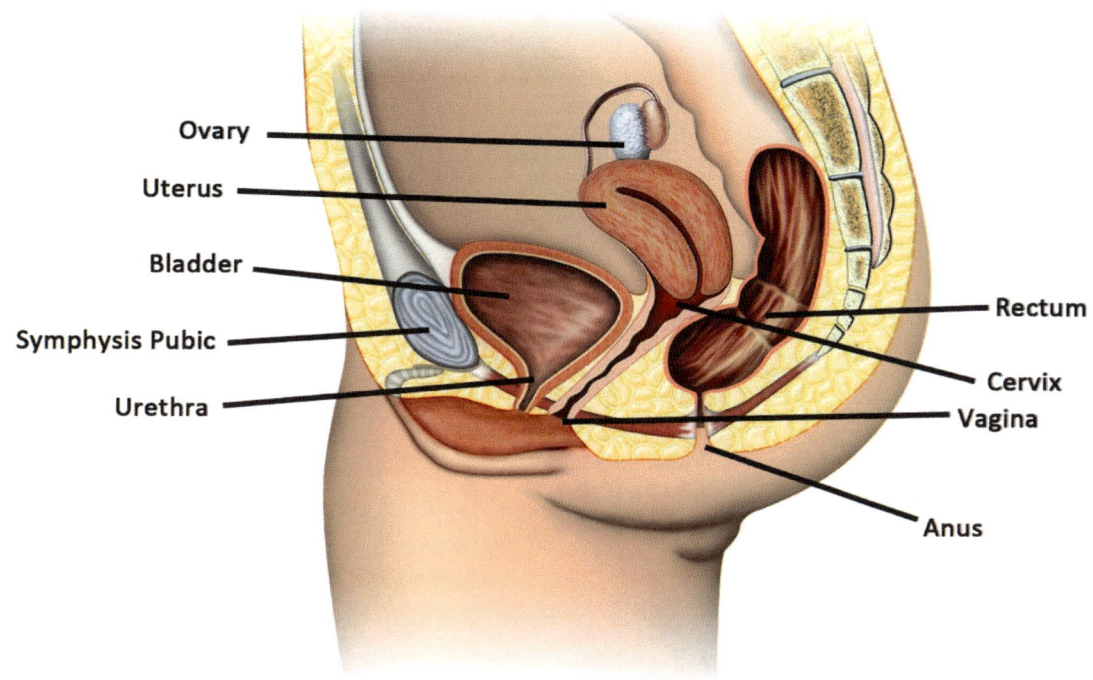

Ovary

Uterus

Bladder

Symphysis Pubic

Urethra

Rectum

Cervix

Vagina

Anus

10

MEDICAL TERMINOLOGY

A. Cardiovascular System

Abdominal Aortic Aneurysm (AAA): when the large main blood vessel that supplies blood to the abdomen, pelvis, and legs becomes abnormally large or balloons outward due to weakness in the arterial wall

AICD: An implantable cardioverter defibrillator; device implanted in the chest wall that detects cardiac arrhythmias and uses electric impulses to correct them. It also has an automatic defibrillator that will correct any dangerous arrhythmias detected.

Aneurysm: Widening/ ballooning of an artery caused by weakness in the arterial wall

Angina: Chest pain caused by decreased blood flow to heart muscle

Aortic dissection: Bleeding along the wall of the aorta, caused by a tear in the aorta.

Arrhythmia: Irregular heartbeat.

Atherosclerosis: Hardening of arteries caused by plaque build-up

Atrial fibrillation (a-fib): Common type of heart arrhythmia which is irregular and often rapid.

Bradycardia: slow heart rate (resting heart rate of < 60 beats per minute).

Bruit: a term used to describe the unusual sound that blood makes when it rushes past an obstruction in an artery.

Capillary refill: A way to measure peripheral perfusion. The amount of time it takes blood to refill empty capillaries. Clinically tested by pressing on finger and seeing how long it takes for color to return.

Cardiac arrest: When the heart stops beating causing normal circulation of blood to stop

Cardiomegaly: enlarged heart

Cardiomyopathy: disease of the heart muscle

Carotid bruit: a systolic murmur heard over the carotid artery in the neck

Congestive heart failure (CHF): Inability of the heart to pump required amount of blood, may cause pulmonary edema

Coronary artery disease (CAD): disease marked by narrowing and hardening of the arteries that supply blood to the heart

Deep vein thrombosis (DVT): blood clot in a deep vein, usually in the lower extremities.

Dysrhythmia: any of a number of disorders marked by abnormal electrical activity in the heart, causing abnormal heart rates and rhythms.

Ectopy: extra heart beats seen on an EKG tracing (PAC, PVC)

Edema: swelling

Ejection fraction (EF): Percentage of blood pumped out of the ventricles with each heartbeat. It is reduced when the heart muscle is damaged and a severe reduction can indicate heart failure.

Rub: an abnormal heart sound, usually a sign of pericarditis.

Gallop: extra abnormal heart sounds heard on a cardiac exam

Hyperlipidemia: High cholesterol (also known as hypercholesterolemia)

Hypertension: High blood pressure.

Hypotension: low blood pressure

Mitral valve prolapse: Occurs when the valve between the heart's left upper chamber (left atrium) and the left lower chamber (left ventricle) doesn't close properly.

Myocardial infarction (MI): "Heart attack", occurs when blood is blocked from going to the heart causing damage to cardiac muscle.

Murmur: sounds produced by turbulent blood flow through the heart valves

Pacemaker: a small device implanted under the skin on the chest wall that uses electrical impulses to correct arrhythmias

Palpitations: sensations of abnormal heart rate including sensation of skipped or extra beats or that the heart is "racing"

Pedal edema: swelling of the feet

Shock: A group of signs and symptoms indicating poor oxygen supply to tissues and insufficient return of blood to the heart.

Stenosis: abnormal narrowing, usually of a blood vessel

Syncope: Fainting

STEMI: ST segment elevation myocardial infarction. A severe heart attack where the coronary artery is completely blocked, causing cardiac muscle damage that results in EKG changes

NSTEMI: Less severe type of MI, which results in less damage to the heart muscle and is noted by the absence of elevated ST segments on an EKG

Tachycardia: fast heart rate (resting heart rate > 100 beats per minute).

Ventricular Hypertrophy: Increase in size of cardiac muscle in the heart's ventricles. Left ventricular hypertrophy (LVH) may be a sign that the heart is working harder to pump blood to the rest of the body.

Wolff-Parkinson-White Syndrome (WPW): condition where there is an abnormal electrical pathway in the heart that leads to periods of a very fast heartbeat (tachycardia). Can be detected on an EKG.

Common Procedures

Cardiac catheterization: A procedure where a catheter is passed into the heart either for diagnostic purposes or intervention to correct a blocked vessel

Coronary Artery Bypass Graft (CABG): a surgical procedure to reroute blood around a diseased section of a coronary artery

Cardiac enzyme test: Measurements of enzymes released into the bloodstream after a heart attack (troponin and myoglobin). Serial measurements can assess whether or not there has been damage to cardiac muscle

Cardiac stent: a procedure that places a mesh tube into a narrowed or blocked coronary artery in effort to open it up

Carotid endarectomy: a surgical procedure to remove plaque in the carotid arteries in an effort to prevent a stroke

Electrocardiogram (EKG/ECG): Measurement of electrical conduction in the heart.

Echocardiogram: Ultrasound of the heart

Holter monitoring: A portable device that records electrical activity in the heart for an extended period of time, usually at least 24 hours, in an effort to detect cardiac arrhythmias.

Stress test: An electrocardiogram plus blood pressure and heart rate measurements shows the heart's response to exertion (exercise stress, nuclear stress).

Cardioversion: Medical procedure using medication or electrical impulse to convert heart rate to a normal sinus rhythm.

B. Respiratory System

Accessory muscle use: condition in which accessory muscles are used to assist with inspiration, a sign of respiratory distress

Apnea: absence of respiration

Asphyxia: Extreme decrease in the amount of oxygen in the body

Asthma: Chronic condition with episodes of inflammation and narrowing of the airways leading to difficulty breathing and wheezing

Atelectasis: partial collapse of lung tissue, seen on a CXR

Bronchitis: inflammation of the air passages between the nose and the lungs, may be acute or chronic

Chronic obstructive pulmonary disease (COPD): common chronic lung disease marked by difficulty breathing; a combination of chronic bronchitis and emphysema

Dyspnea: difficulty breathing

Dyspnea on exertion (DOE): Shortness of breath worsened with mild exertion

Emphysema: Hyperinflation of air sacs with destruction of alveolar walls.

Hemoptysis: coughing up blood

Hemothorax: blood in the pleural cavity

Hypoxia: reduced oxygen supply to tissue

Pneumonia: Infection of the lung

Pulmonary embolism (PE): obstruction of blood vessel in the lungs, usually due to a blood clot

Pneumothorax: collapsed lung

Rales: crackling noises heard on auscultation of the lung during inhalation

Respiratory distress: the inability to adequately ventilate causing physically labored ventilation

Retractions: inward movement of the chest wall with inspiration; usually a sign of respiratory distress

Rhonchi: coarse rattling breath sound

Sputum: mucus coughed up from the airways

Stridor: a wheeze-like sound heard on auscultation, usually a sign of an obstructed airway

Tuberculosis: An infectious disease caused by bacteria.

Tachypnea: Increased respiratory rate

Wheezes: course, whistling lung sound caused by narrowed airways

Common Procedures

Endotracheal intubation: A tube is placed through the nose or mouth into the trachea to establish an airway

Tracheostomy: Creation of an opening into the trachea through the neck and the insertion of a tube to create an airway.

C. HEENT

Anisocoria: unequal pupil sizes

Cerumen: Earwax

Conjunctivitis: Inflammation of the conjunctiva.

Diplopia: double vision

Dentition: the arrangement of teeth

Dental caries: Tooth decay

Epistaxis: nosebleed

Extra ocular movements (EOM): Movements of the eyes controlled by six muscles

Fontanel: soft spot on an infant's skull

Hemotympanum: presence of blood in the tympanic cavity of the ear, usually a sign of skull fracture as a result of trauma

Icterus: jaundice (yellowing) seen in the sclera (white part) of the eye

Injected conjunctiva: redness of the sclera, sign of conjunctivitis

Malocclusion: misalignment of the teeth

Nares: external openings of the nasal canal (nostrils)

Nasal septal hematoma: accumulation of blood within the nasal septum, usually a result of trauma

Nystagmus: rapid involuntary eye movements (can be horizontal, vertical, or rotary)

Occiput: referring to the occipital area of the skull (lower back region of the head)

Pharyngeal erythema: redness of the throat

Pharyngitis: inflammation of the pharynx

Pale conjunctivae: paleness of the conjunctiva, often seen in anemic patients

Papilledema: swelling of the optic disc, sign of increased cranial pressure

Photophobia: sensitivity and aversion to light due to discomfort or pain to the eyes with light exposure

Rhinorrhea: runny nose

Strabismus: improper alignment of the eyes

Sty (stye): Pus-filled (purulent) infection of glands near the eyelid

Subconjunctival hemorrhage: bleeding that occurs underneath the conjunctiva, seen as a bright red patch on the sclera

Tinnitus: Abnormal (ringing, buzzing, roaring) sound in the ears.

Tonsillar exudates: grayish-white coating on the tonsillar surface

Trismus: inability to open the mouth fully

Upper respiratory infection (URI): nonspecific infection in the upper respiratory tract

Zygoma: delicate facial bone, often a site of injury in assaults

D. Endocrine System

Adenoidectomy: surgical excision of the adenoids

Addison's Disease: Adrenal gland disorder

Diabetes mellitus (DM): A disorder of the pancreas that causes an increase in blood glucose levels.

Diabetic ketoacidosis (DKA): complication of diabetes that occurs when the body cannot use glucose so it begins to burn fatty acids; forming ketone bodies as by-products. The large accumulation of ketones causes metabolic acidosis, which distinguishes this diabetic complication from others.

Goiter: Enlargement of the thyroid gland.

Gout: form of arthritis caused by uric acid buildup in the joints

Hyperthyroidism: Over-activity of the thyroid gland.

Hypothyroidism: under activity of the thyroid gland

Thyromegaly: abnormally enlarged thyroid gland

E. Gastrointestinal System

Appendicitis: A condition in which the appendix becomes inflamed

Abdominal distention: swelling or enlargement of the abdomen

Ascites: accumulation of fluid in the abdominal cavity

Bowel sounds: a physical exam finding, may be hypoactive or hyperactive

C-difficile: ("c.diff") a bacteria in the intestines, which causes diarrhea and GI upset, usually a side effect of antibiotic use.

Cholelithiasis: Gallstones

Cholecystitis: inflammation of the gallbladder, clinically may present as RUQ tenderness

Cirrhosis: Chronic degenerative liver disease

Crohn's Disease: a form of inflammatory bowel disease

Decreased rectal tone: damage to the muscles that surround the rectum

Diverticulosis: Condition where there is small abnormal pouches (diverticula) in the intestinal wall

Diverticulitis: Inflammation and infection within the diverticula.

Dyspepsia: Indigestion

Emesis: vomiting

Gastroesophageal reflux disease (GERD): A condition in which contents of the stomach flow back into the esophagus, known as "reflux"

Gastrointestinal (GI) bleed: any bleeding in the gastrointestinal tract, usually classified as "upper" or "lower" GI bleed

Gravid uterus: a uterus containing a developing fetus

Guarding: contraction of abdominal muscles and discomfort when pressure is applied to the abdomen

GUAIAC test: a diagnostic test looking for occult blood in the stool. It is done after taking a small stool sample during a rectal examination

Hepatomegaly: increased size of the liver

Hepatitis: Inflammation of the liver.

Hematemesis: Vomiting of blood

Hematochezia: passage of bright red blood in the stool

Hemorrhoids: painful, swollen veins in the anus or rectum. May be internal or external and cause rectal bleeding

Ileus: partial or complete bowel obstruction

Irritable Bowel Syndrome (IBS): A common disorder that affects the large intestine (colon). Commonly causes cramping, abdominal pain, bloating gas, diarrhea and constipation.

Jaundice: Yellow coloration of the skin/mucus membranes from high levels of bilirubin in the bloodstream

McBurney's point tenderness: a site of extreme sensitivity in acute appendicitis, situated in the normal area of the appendix midway between the umbilicus and the anterior iliac crest in the right lower quadrant

Melena: black "tarry" colored stool, a sign of GI bleeding

Murphy's Sign: A test looking for acute cholecystitis where there is increased tenderness in the RUQ when it is palpated upon expiration.

Organomegaly: abnormal enlargement of an organ

Pancreatitis: inflammation of the pancreas

Rebound: an increase in severe pain and discomfort when pressure is abruptly relieved from localized region of the abdomen.

Rigid: hardness/stiffening of the abdomen

Rovsing's sign: indication of acute appendicitis in which pressure on the LLQ of the abdomen causes pain in the RLQ.

Small bowel obstruction (SBO): any obstruction in the intestines, may be full or partial, also known as an ileus

Splenomegaly: abnormal enlargement of the spleen

Common Procedures

Appendectomy: surgery to remove the appendix

Colectomy: a surgical procedure to remove all or part of your colon

Liver function tests (LFTs): Measurements of liver enzymes and other substances in the blood. Enzyme levels increase when the liver is damaged (as in hepatitis).

Cholecystectomy: surgical removal of the gallbladder

Colonoscopy: internal examination of the colon using a small camera

F. Genitourinary System

Amenorrhea: Absence of menstrual flow

Adnexal tenderness: findings of tenderness in the ovarian region of females during a bi-manual exam

Benign Prostatic Hypertrophy/ hyperplasia (BPH): A condition where the prostate is enlarged, may cause difficulty with urination

Cervical dilation: opening of the cervix

Cervical motion tenderness: finding of tenderness on a pelvic exam, which suggests pelvic etiology, classically found in PID

Costovertebral Angle (CVA) tenderness: physical exam finding suggestive of renal etiology

Cervicitis: inflammation of the cervix

Dyspareunia: painful sexual intercourse

Dysmenorrhea: Painful menstrual flow

Dysuria: painful urination

Ectopic pregnancy: pregnancy complication that occurs when the fertilized ovum is implanted in any tissue other than the uterine wall

Endometriosis: condition where cells from the lining of the uterus grow in other areas of the body.

Flank pain: pain on the side of the body between the abdomen and back, often indicative of renal pathology

GPA (Grava/Para/Abortus): total number of pregnancies, number of live births, number of births terminated or miscarried

Hematuria: blood in the urine

Hemodialysis: a method for removing waste products from the blood in individuals with advanced renal disease

Inguinal: relating to the groin

Nephrolithiasis: kidney stones

Polyuria: excessive urination

Prostatitis: Inflammation of the prostate gland, often requires antibiotic treatment

Pyelonephritis: a kidney infection caused by a progressive urinary tract infection

LMP: last menstrual period

Menorrhagia: heavy menstrual bleeding

Renal insufficiency: (renal failure) Loss of kidney function, may be either acute or chronic

Urinary tract infection (UTI): bacterial infection in the urinary tract

Urinary incontinence: Involuntary leakage of urine

Ureterolithiasis: kidney stones that have progressed to the ureter

Common Procedures

Tubal ligation: a surgical procedure done to permanently sterilize a female by blocking or severing the fallopian tubes, also known as "tying tubes"

D&C (dilation & curettage): a procedure in which the cervix is dilated and part of the inner lining of the uterus and/or contents of the uterus are surgically removed

Cesarean section (c-section): surgical delivery of an infant

Hysterectomy: surgical removal of the uterus and/or ovaries

Nephrectomy: surgical removal of a kidney

G. Musculoskeletal System

Arthralgia: joint pain

Avulsion: an injury where a structure is torn off of another. An avulsion fracture may occur when a ligament tears and pulls a bone fragment off with it

Dislocation: abnormal separation of two bones at a joint

Fracture: A break in a bone, may be displaced (out of alignment) or non-displaced

Joint effusion: swollen joint

Malleolus: bony structure on either side of the ankle, common site of fracture

Myalgia: muscle pain

Rhabdomyolysis: "rhabdo" condition where skeletal muscle breaks down quickly and releases toxins.

Sprain: Ligamentous injury caused by the ligament being stretched beyond its capacity causing pain and swelling to the joint

Strain: an injury to the muscle where it is either torn r stretched beyond its capacity

H. Neck / Back

Cauda equina syndrome: serious condition where the terminal portion of the spinal cord is compressed. If left untreated can lead to permanent loss of bowel/bladder function as well as lower extremity paralysis

C-collar: A neck brace that is put in place after a trauma and possible neck injury. It is removed after either exam or radiographic imaging has assured there is no c-spine injury

Cervical: pertaining to the neck

Cervical lymphadenopathy: swollen lymph nodes in the neck

CVA tenderness: costovertebral angle tenderness, usually dues to a kidney disease

Jugular Venous Distension (JVD): swelling/distension of the jugular vein due to elevated blood pressure in the vein.

Meningismus: neck stiffness (nuchal rigidity)

Nuchal: pertaining to the neck region

Paraspinal: pain that is lateral to the spine, it is suggestive of a muscular etiology

Sciatica: pain, weakness, numbness or tingling in the leg caused by compression of the sciatic nerve

Supple: easily movable without pain

Thyromegaly: enlarged thyroid

Vertebral point tenderness: tenderness over the midline of the back on the vertebrae

I. Nervous System

Aphasia: general term referring to any impairment in speech ability

Ataxia: Lack of muscle movement coordination

Babinski reflex: A reflex that occurs when the toes fan outward in response to the bottom of the foot being stimulated. This is normal in infants under the age of 2, however if present in adults may be a sign of a neurologic disorder.

Bell's palsy: unilateral paralysis of the facial muscles supplied by cranial nerve VII

Cerebrospinal fluid (CSF): Fluid surrounding the brain and spinal cord, samples of this are taken during a lumbar puncture to look for infection

Central nervous system (CNS): The part of the nervous system containing the brain and spinal cord

Cerebrovascular accident (CVA): Stroke. Any interruption of blood supply to the brain; caused by either a blood clot in a cerebral artery (ischemic stroke) or a burst blood vessel (hemorrhagic stroke).

Clonus: series of rapid repeated muscle contractions and relaxations

Concussion: A type of TBI that causes some temporary loss of neurologic function.

Dementia: General term for a variety of neurologic disorders that result in a loss of cognitive function

Dysarthria: difficulty speaking due to loss of control over the muscles controlling the mouth and face

Dysdiadochokinesia: Inability to perform rapid alternating movement test

Epilepsy: A condition in which a person has recurrent seizures

Finger to nose test: test of coordination in which the patient is asked to touch their nose with their finger and then touch the physician's finger and then to touch their nose again.

Gait: a manner of walking, abnormalities can indicate a variety of neurologic disorders

Heel to shin test: A neurologic test testing lower limb coordination and position sense

Hemiparesis: weakness on one side of the body

Hemiplegia: complete paralysis of one side of the body

Lumbar puncture (LP): "spinal tap"

Meningitis: Inflammation of the meninges (membranes surrounding the brain and spinal cord)

Parethesia: altered skin sensation such as "burning", "prickling" or "tingling"

Straight-leg raise test: test often performed to determine whether a patient with low back pain has an underlying herniated disk

Pronator drift: neurologic test where a patient stand with arms outstretched and eyes closed. A drift occurs when the patient's arm has a tendency to pronate in this position

Romberg test: test of coordination in which the patient is asked to stand with their feet together and eyes closed. Abnormal tests occur when a patient falls or sways to one side consistently.

Radiculopathy: A condition where there is pain or altered sensation along the path of a compressed nerve

Transient ischemic accident (TIA): Temporary loss of blood flow to an area of the brain, resulting in short term stroke-like symptoms

Traumatic brain injury (TBI): Damage to the brain as the result of an injury, can cause a variety of neurologic symptoms

J. Integumentary (Skin)

Cellulitis: skin infection

Cyanosis: bluish color to the skin or mucus membranes due to a lack of oxygen in the blood.

Contusion: bruise

Decubitus ulcer: pressure ulcer, also known as a "bed sore"

Debridement: removal of infected or dead tissue from a wound to promote healing of healthy tissue

Dehiscence: reopening of a previously closed wound

Dermatitis: inflammation of the skin

Diaphoresis: sweating

Dysphagia: difficulty swallowing

Ecchymosis: bruising

Erythema: redness

Hematoma: bruise

Hyperkalemia: high potassium

Hypernatremia: high sodium

Hypercalcemia: high calcium

Induration: an abnormally hard area overlying an area of soft tissue or organ

Keloid: abnormal scar formation

Pallor: paleness

Paronychia: skin infection that occurs around the nails

Petechia: tiny red spots on the skin

Poor skin turgor: sign of dehydration

Psoriasis: common skin condition marked by dry, scaly patches and itching

Purulent: having pus

Pruitic: itchy

Urticaria: hives

K. Kinesiology

Abduction: draws away from the midline

Adduction: draws toward the midline

Anatomical position: to stand erect with arms at sides and palms turned forward

Anterior: situated in front of or directed toward the front

Deep: farther from the surface

Distal: farther from the limb root

Extension: straightening out

External: outside

Flexion: bending or angulation

Frontal: divides the body into anterior and posterior parts

Lateral: farther from the midline

Medial: nearer to the midline

Midline: divides the body into right and left

Palmar: palm side of the hand or body

Plantar: sole side of foot

Posterior: rear or back

Pronate: that which turns palm of hand downward

Prone: face down

Proximal: nearer to the limb root

Superficial: nearer to the surface

Superior: upper, nearer to the crown

Supinate: that which turns palm of hand upward

Supine: body lying face up

Transverse: right angles to long axis; divides body into upper and lower parts

L. Psychiatric

Anxiety: Feeling of apprehension or worry, may cause physical symptoms such as headaches, sweats or nausea

Depression: ongoing feeling of sadness or low mood, which interferes with activities of daily living

Flat Affect: reduction or complete loss of emotional expression

Hallucinations: sensory perception in the absence of an actual sensory stimulus; may be auditory, visual or tactile

Insomnia: Difficulty falling asleep or staying asleep

Psychosis: Loss of concept of reality, may be a side affect of a medication or symptom of an underlying disease

Suicidal Ideation: medical term for having thoughts of suicide, which may include having a specific suicidal plan

M. Other Miscellaneous Terms

Ambulatory: able to walk

Anemia: general term for a variety of disorders in which the body does not have enough healthy red blood cells carrying oxygen in the body

Anasarca: extensive sub-q edema

Afebrile: without fever

Axilla: armpit

Crepitus: cracking/crunching sound produced when the ends of a fractured piece of bone rub against each other or by air moving into tissue space

Cachectic: physical appearance of loss of weight and muscle wasting seen in patients with advanced stages of diseases such as cancer or AIDs

Emaciated: appearing extremely thin due to loss of fat tissue and muscle mass

Etiology: the cause of a symptom

Febrile: feverish

Hemorrhage: heavy bleeding

Infiltrate: abnormal collection within a tissue or cell; often how pneumonia is described on a CXR

Leukocytosis: elevated WBC

Lymphadenopathy: abnormally enlarged lymph nodes

Lymphangitis: infection and inflammation of the lymph vessels

Malaise: general feeling of illness

Mastectomy: surgical removal of the breast

Somnolent: "drowsy" or sleepy appearance

Sepsis: severe bacterial blood infection, the infection usually begins at another site and travels to the blood

Torsion: twisting of an organ (i.e. testicular torsion)

Vertigo: A type of dizziness that gives the sensation that the room is "spinning" or moving when one is standing still

11

COMMON DIAGNOSTIC TESTS

Blood Tests

Basic Metabolic Panel (BMP): Includes glucose, Ca, electrolytes (Na, K, CO_2, Cl), kidney function tests (BUN/creatinine)

Complete blood count (CBC): Looks at blood counts to assess for infection, anemia or other conditions.

Comprehensive Metabolic Panel (CMP): Includes 14 different tests to evaluate the current status of your kidneys, liver, electrolytes and acid/base balance as well as blood sugar and blood proteins

B-type natriuric protein (BNP): used to assess for CHF

Cardiac enzymes: Troponin and CK-MB (creatine kinase)

Type & Screen: Looks at a blood type and screens for antibodies, used if a blood transfusion is needed

B-HCG: Blood test measuring levels of the pregnancy hormone

Stool cultures: Looks for bacterial or parasitic causes of diarrhea

Fibrinogen D-dimer (d-dimer): blood test used to screen for possible blood clot

INR / PTT / PT: Blood tests used to assess the tendency of blood to clot. This is important to check in patients who are on anti-coagulant medications to be sure they are within a therapeutic range

Thyroid function tests: TSH/T4

Lactic Acid: measured to assess for severe sepsis

Liver function tests (LFTs) / Hepatic function panel: tests that assess for liver damage

Urinalysis: Analysis of the urine to look for UTI or kidney disease

Radiology

Ultrasound (US): a diagnostic test that uses high frequency sound waves to see body structures in real time. The benefit of the test is that it does not use radiation. It does have some limitations in that the waves do not travel well through adipose tissue or gas which makes observing the abdomen and bowel difficult at times.

Doppler US: A special type of US that allows blood flow to be seen. This test is used to diagnose DVTs and testicular/ovarian torsions for example.

CT scan: combines a series of x-ray views taken from many different angles to produce cross-sectional images of the bones and soft tissues inside your body. There are many types of CT scans used, which are based on what the physician is looking for. The drawbacks of a CT scan are the high levels of radiation used and the limitations in use with patients who have renal failure. These patients cannot have contrast CT scans because their kidneys cannot clear the contrast. In addition, CT scans expose patients to radiation, and over time repeated exposure may lead to cancer.

Common CT scans include:
- CT head: looks for stroke, occult skull fracture
- CT spine (C,T, L,S): looks for injury after trauma
- CT abdomen/pelvis without contrast: used to look for kidney stone
- CT abdomen/pelvis with contrast: used to assess for abdominal pathology
- CT chest: looks for aortic dissection or PE

X-ray (XR): known as "plane x-rays", a type of radiologic study that uses electromagnetic radiation to look at the body. Limitations are that it does not allow soft tissues or organs to be well visualized.

Common XRs include:

- Bone XR: look at bones to assess for fracture or dislocation
- Chest x-ray (CXR): Looks for pneumonia, pneumothorax, cardiomegaly, and other lung abnormalities
- Abdominal XR: looks for bowel obstruction (ileus)
- XR KUB: Looks at the kidneys, ureters and bladder for renal stones. Usually these are not well visualized on XR and other diagnostic tests may be needed.

MRI: magnetic resonance imaging: technique that uses a magnetic field and radio waves to create detailed images of the organs and tissues within the body. Drawbacks of using this type of imaging include the large cost associated with MRIs, and the amount of time the test takes (approximately 1 hour per body part imaged). This is often not readily available in an emergency department and patients may need to be admitted for MRIs if needed on an emergent basis.

HIDA: A nuclear imaging test that looks at the flow of bile from the liver to the small intestines. It is used to evaluate the gallbladder and bile ducts. This is usually done to evaluate RUQ pain if a patient has a negative CT scan and gallbladder etiology is still suspected.

12

MEDICAL ABBREVIATIONS

ASA: Aspirin

ACS: Acute coronary syndrome

AAA: abdominal aortic aneurysm

ABG: arterial blood gas

ABx: antibiotics

AICD: automatic implantable cardioverter defibrillator

AKA: above the knee amputation

AMA: Against Medical Advice

AMS: altered mental status

ANS: autonomic nervous system

A&O x (1,2,3,4): alert and oriented x… (1-person, 2-place, 3-time, 4- event)

Appy: appendectomy

B: bilateral

BID: 2 times/day

BKA: below the knee amputation

BM: bowel movement

BP: blood pressure

BUN: blood urea nitrogen

C-spine: cervical spine

CA: cancer

Ca: calcium

CAD: coronary artery disease

CBC: complete blood count

CC: chief complaint

CF: cystic fibrosis

CHF: congestive heart failure

CNS: central nervous system

c/o: complaining of

COPD: chronic obstructive pulmonary disease

CSF: cerebrospinal fluid

CTA: clear to auscultation

CVA: cerebrovascular accident or costal vertebral angle

CXR: chest x-ray

D&C: dilation/curettage

DKA: diabetic ketoacidosis

DM: diabetes mellitus

DTs: delirium tremens (seen in ETOH withdrawal)

DTR: deep tendon reflex

Dx: diagnosis

ECG / EKG: electrocardiogram

EEG: electroencephalo- gram/-graph

ENT: ear, nose, throat

ETOH: alcohol

FB: foreign body

FFP: fresh frozen plasma

ESRD: end stage renal disease

FROM: full range of motion

GB: gallbladder

GERD: gastro esophageal reflux disease

GI: gastrointestinal

GSW: gunshot wound

GYN: gynecology

HA: headache

HEENT: head, ears, eyes, nose, throat

h/o: history of

HR: heart rate

HTN: hypertension

IDDM: insulin dependent diabetes mellitus

NIDDM: non-insulin dependent diabetes mellitus

IM: intramuscular

IUD: intrauterine device

IV: intravenous

JVD: jugular vein distension

K: potassium

KUB: kidney, ureter, bladder

L: left

LBBB: left bundle branch block

LFT: liver function test

LE: Lower extremity

LQ: Lower quadrant

LOC: loss of consciousness

LMP: last menstrual period

LP: lumbar puncture

LUL: left upper lobe (of the lung)

LLL: left lower lobe (of the lung)

L-spine: lumbar spine

LS-spine: lumbosacral spine

LVH: left ventricular hypertrophy

(A)MI: (acute) myocardial infarction

MVA / MVC: Motor vehicle accident / crash

NAD: no acute distress

NADP (NAD): No acute disease process/ no acute disease

NKA / NKDA: no known allergies/ no known drug allergies

NPO: nothing by mouth (no food/drink)

NSR: normal sinus rhythm

NTG: nitroglycerine

NVID: neurovascularly intact distally

O2: oxygen

OM: otitis media

OE: otitis externa

Ortho: orthopedics

OT: occupational therapy

PAC: premature atrial contraction

PCP: primary care physician

PMD: primary medical doctor

PO: "Per os", by mouth

PE: pulmonary embolism

PEx: physical exam

PERRLA: pupils equal, round, regular, react to light, accommodate

PID: pelvic inflammatory disease

PNS: peripheral nervous system

PO: by mouth

PRN: as needed

PT: physical therapy

Pt: patient

PTA: prior to arrival

PVC: premature ventricular contraction

PVD: peripheral vascular disease

QID: 4 times/day

QH: every hour

Q4H or q4: every 4 hours

R: right

RBC: red blood cell

r/o: rule out

ROM: range of motion

ROS: review of systems

RR: respiration rate

RBBB: right bundle branch block

RXN: reaction

SBO: small bowel obstruction

TID: 3 times/day

T-spine: thoracic spine

TMJ: temporomandibular joint

Fx: fracture

Hx: history

Rx: prescription

Sx: symptoms

SVT: Supraventricular tachycardia

RVR: rapid ventricular rate

Tx: treatment

UE: Upper extremity

UQ: Upper quadrant

sub q: subcutaneous

SOB: shortness of breath

s/p: status post

STAT: immediately

SVT: supraventricular tachycardia

TIA: transient ischemic attack

TM: tympanic membrane

UA: urine analysis

US: ultrasound

UTI: urinary tract infection

VS: vital signs

VSS: vital signs stable

WBC: white blood count

WNL: within normal limits

WPW: Wolff-Parkinson-White syndrome

XR: x-ray

Y/O: years old

13

COMMON MEDICATIONS IN THE EMERGENCY ROOM

A. Analgesics

- Acetaminophen (Tylenol)

NSAIDS:

- Ibuprofen (Motrin)

- ASA

- Naproxen (Aleve, Naprosyn)

- Toradol (Keterolac)

Narcotics:

- Percocet

- Darvocet

- Vicodin

- Morphine

- Dilaudid

B. Antibiotics

- Amoxicillin

- Ampicillin

- Augmentin

B. Antibiotics (Cont.)

- Azithromycin

- Bactrim

- Cephalexin (Keflex)

- Ciprofloxacin (Cipro)

- Clindamycin

- Ceftriaxone

- Doxycycline

- Erythromycin

- Flagyl

- Levaquin

- Penicillin

- Rocephin

- Tobramycin

- Unasyn

- Vancomycin

C. Antiemetics (anti-nausea)

- Compazine

- Phenergan

- Zofran

D. Respiratory/ Allergy Medications

- Albuterol: sometimes referred to as a nebulizer

- Epinephrine: used to stimulate heart or control anaphylaxis

- Solumedrol: long acting corticosteroid given to prevent anaphylaxis and in asthma patients

- Prednisone: corticosteroid

- Benadryl: allergy medication

E. Cardiac Medications

Anti-coagulants:

- Warfarin (Coumadin)

- ASA

- Heparin

- Lovenox

- tPA

- Plavix

Cholesterol Medications:

- Simvastatin

- Lipitor

Diuretics:

- Lasix

- Bumex (furosemide)

F. Other GI Medications

- Prevacid: used to treat GERD and ulcers

- Omeprazole (Prilosec): used to treat GERD and ulcers

- Pepcid: antacid

- GI cocktail: mixture of medications used to treat GI upset

G. Miscellaneous Medications

- **Ativan (Lorazepam):** Used to treat anxiety and alcohol withdrawal, in the class of drugs called benzodiazepines ("benzos")

- **Depakote:** used to treat seizure disorders and mood disorders (bipolar disorder)

- **Valproic Acid:** used to treat seizure disorders, may see toxicity in an emergency setting if a patient has taken too much

- **Keppra:** Used to treat epilepsy

- **Klonopin:** A benzo used to treat seizure disorders and panic attacks

- **Neurontin:** Used to prevent and control seizures, also used to relieve nerve pain such as pain during shingles

- **Dilantin:** anticonvulsant

- **Phenobarbital:** sedative/ anticonvulsant

- **Xanax:** a type of benzo, used to treat anxiety

- **Valium (Diazepam):** powerful sedative / anti-convulsant

- **Versed:** type of powerful, short-acting sedative often used in conscious sedations for procedures in the ED

- **Lidocaine:** local anesthetic

- **Fluorescein:** a dye used in eye exams to stain the cornea and look for abrasions

- **Haldol:** sedative/anti-psychotic

14

COMMON CLINICAL SCENARIOS

The following are common chief complaints that you may encounter. Below each are some factors you should be thinking about and taking into consideration when charting the HPI on these patients. The physician will guide the questioning, but it will be helpful for you to be able to anticipate the questions and taking history, as you are in the room.

1. Abdominal Pain

a. Location is important: RUQ, RLQ, LUQ, LLQ, Epigastric, flank
b. Associated symptoms: fever, nausea, vomiting, diarrhea, vaginal bleeding or discharge, hematuria, dysuria
c. Medical/Surgical/ Familial history: Has the patient had any abdominal surgeries? Does the patient have a h/o ovarian cysts? Does the patient have family h/o gallstones?
d. If the patient has diarrhea: have they had any recent antibiotic use, travel out of the country, contaminated food exposure?
e. Is there any blood in the emesis or stool? Is there black tarry stool (melena)?

2. Chest Pain

a. Location/ radiation
b. Associated features: diaphoresis, dyspnea, nausea, dizziness (this is especially important because women present with very different cardiac symptoms than men)
c. Is the pain worse with exertion? Is it only with deep breathing (pleuritic)?
d. PE risk factors: birth control, recent travel with prolonged immobility, smoking, recent surgery, h/o cancer, calf swelling or tenderness, personal or familial h/o clots or clotting disorders
e. Is the pain associated with fever/ cough? Is the cough productive? (possible pneumonia)
f. Is the pain reproducible with palpation? (likely musculoskeletal)
g. If a person is being admitted for unstable angina, must document certain EKG findings.

3. Injuries

 a. What type of injury? Fall, contact sport, head injury, extremity injury, MVC?
 b. Is the patient on anticoagulants?
 c. Are there any other injuries in addition to the main injury? (If there is a major source of pain other secondary injuries may be overlooked.)
 d. In a head injury/fall: was there LOC? Has the person been acting normally since? Are there any neurologic deficits?
 e. MVC: Was the patient a driver or passenger? What was the mechanism of the accident (speed, point of impact, amount of damage to car)? Was the patient restrained? Did airbags deploy?
 f. In a fall, was it a mechanical fall or were there any preceding symptoms?
 g. In musculoskeletal injuries: is the sensation intact around the injury?

4. Headache

 a. Did the headache come on suddenly?
 b. Is it the "worst headache of their life"? (This will usually warrant a head CT so be careful about documenting this)
 c. Have they had headaches like this in the past?
 d. Have there been any fevers, neck stiffness, or photophobia? (Clinician may be thinking possibly meningitis and may perform an LP)

5. Stroke like symptoms

 a. When was the onset of the symptoms?
 b. How long did the symptoms last? (These are both important questions to ask because tPA can only be given within a certain time frame)
 c. Were the symptoms one sided?
 d. Were the symptoms precipitated by a headache?
 e. Does the patient have a h/o HTN or TIAs?

6. Bleeding or pain during pregnancy

    a.   When was the patient's LMP?

    b.   What is the patient's pregnancy history? (G/P/AB)

    c.   Does the patient smoke or drink?

7. Mental Health Evaluation

    a.   Is the person suicidal or homicidal?

    b.   Do they have a specific plan?

    c.   Do they have a h/o prior suicide attempts or psychiatric admissions?

Other

    a. For pediatric cases, never document that a child is "lethargic"

    b. When documenting oxygen saturation, be sure to note if the patient is on oxygen and how much

15

PRACTICE CLINICAL SCENARIO SCRIPTS

Scenario #1: Abdominal Pain

Doctor: "What brings you to the emergency room today?"

Patient: "Well, I have this horrible abdominal pain on the upper right side of my stomach."

Doctor: "How long have you had this pain for?"

Patient: "Well it started Monday, and I haven't had it the whole time but after dinner today it got way worse and I threw up, so I came here."

Doctor: "Ok, so you've had this pain on and off for 5 days now. What did you have for dinner today?"

Patient: "Some chicken and salad. Oh, it hurts so bad! I think I need some medicine."

Doctor: "Ok, we'll get you something for that in a second, I need to get the rest of your story first. Have you noticed the pain has gotten worse every time you eat?"

Patient: "I'm not sure, maybe sometimes…"

Doctor: "Ok. How would you describe the pain? Is it sharp, dull, crampy…?"

Patient: "It's always kind of there, but when it gets bad it feels kind of sharp, like a knife stabbing."

Doctor: "Ok, now you mentioned that you vomited today, was this the first time you vomited with this pain?"

Patient: "Well, I felt nauseous before, but today was the only time I vomited."

Doctor: "Was there any blood in the vomit, or was it coffee ground colored?"

Patient: "No, it was my dinner."

Doctor: "Alright, we'll get you something for the pain and nausea as soon as I finish examining you. I'm going to ask you some more questions about your health recently. Have you had any fevers or chills?"

Patient: "No."

Doctor: "Recent cough, sore throat, runny nose…?"

Patient: "No."

Doctor: "How about any pain when you urinate, or blood in your urine?"

Patient: "No."

Doctor: "Any chest pain, shortness of breath, rash, or headache?"

Patient: "No."

Doctor: "Alright good, any chance you may be pregnant?"

Patient: "No, my period started 2 days ago."

Doctor: "Ok. Do you have any other medical problems I should know about?"

Patient: "I have asthma, but I haven't had an attack in years. And I had my tonsils out when I was 11."

Doctor: "Alright, have you had any abdominal surgeries?"

Patient: "Just a C-section."

Doctor: "Alright, do you smoke or drink?"

Patient: "I have a glass of wine occasionally but that's all."

Doctor: "Alright, let me just examine your abdomen and then we'll get you that medication."

CC: _____

HPI: _____

_____

_____

_____

_____

ROS: _____

_____

_____

_____

_____

Past medical / surgical / social history:_____

_____

_____

CC: Abdominal Pain

HPI: 34 y/o female presents to emergency complaining of upper right quadrant abdominal pain that began 5 days ago. The pain is intermittent and described as a "stabbing" pain. The pain is associated with nausea and after the patient's dinner tonight of fried chicken and salad, she had one episode of emesis. No hematemesis. LNMP began 2 days ago. No fever, chills, cough, sore throat, congestion, urinary symptoms or chest pain. No other complaints or modifying factors.

ROS:

Positive for: RUQ abdominal pain, nausea, vomiting

Negative for: diarrhea, chills, fever, dysuria, hematuria, cough, sore throat, chest pain, rash, headache, shortness of breath

Past medical / surgical / social history: Pt has h/o asthma, tonsillectomy, c-section. LMP 2 days ago. Pt is a non-smoker. Drinks wine occasionally.

Scenario #2: Motor Vehicle Accident

Doctor: "Hello, I understand you were in a car accident. Tell me what happened."

Patient: "I was turning left out of the mall and a car came out of nowhere and hit me. I hit my head on something, I think? Am I bleeding?"

Doctor: "It looks like you have a superficial scrape, but we'll look at that in a second. Were you wearing a seatbelt?"

Patient: "Yes, I had my seatbelt on and the airbags went off."

Doctor: "Alright. When you hit your head did you lose consciousness?"

Patient: "No, I don't think so."

Doctor: "How fast were you and the other car going? Where did the car hit you?"

Patient: "Well, I was just pulling out, so not too fast. But the speed limit on the road is 45, so the other car must have been going about that speed or faster. I don't know, it all happened so fast! The car hit right behind my door and my car spun around."

Doctor: "Were you able to get up and walk at the scene?"

Patient: "I got up out of the car, but when the ambulance came they made me lay down."

Doctor: "Alright, besides the cut, does anything else hurt? Arms, legs, neck, back?"

Patient: "Well my neck hurts a little, and my left arm hurts."

Doctor: "Alright, we'll keep you in the c-collar then until we get some pictures of your neck. Can you move your arms and legs?"

Patient: "Yeah, I think. Ouch, my left arm hurts to move it."

Doctor: "Alright does your belly hurt at all?"

Patient: "No."

Doctor: "A few more questions… have you had any recent illness with cough, runny nose, pain urinating, shortness of breath, fever, nausea, vomiting, or diarrhea?"

Patient: "No, I've been healthy."

Doctor: "Alright, I'm going to get a CT of your head and neck just to be sure you don't have any internal injuries there. You have some bruising on your left upper arm, so we'll get an x-ray of that arm to be sure it isn't broken. Do you need anything for pain?"

Patient: "Yes, please."

Doctor: "Do you have someone to drive you home?"

Patient: "Yeah, my girlfriend is on her way here."

Doctor: "Alright, a couple more questions… Do you smoke or drink?"

Patient: "I smoke."

Doctor: "How much?"

Patient: "Like a half pack a day. I'm trying to quit."

Doctor: "Alright, keep trying to quit! Any other health problems or surgeries?"

Patient: "No, nothing else."

CC: _____

HPI: _____

_____

_____

_____

_____

ROS: _____

_____

_____

_____

_____

Past medical / surgical / social history:_____

_____

_____

CC: MVC

HPI: 23 y/o male, with no significant past medical history, presents to emergency with head, neck and left arm pain s/p MVC. The patient was a restrained driver turning left when a car going ~45 mph t-boned his driver's side passenger door. The air bags did deploy and the patient states he hit his head but denies LOC. He was able to ambulate immediately following the accident. Currently he states he has neck pain and left arm pain. Left arm pain is exacerbated by movement. No headache, vision changes, chest pain, abdominal pain, SOB, dyspnea, abdominal pain, urinary symptoms, fever or chills. Pt is currently in a c-collar. No other complaints or modifying factors at this time.

ROS: Positive for ecchymosis, arm pain, neck pain, head laceration.

Negative for abdominal pain, chest pain, LOC, headache, dysuria, SOB, rhinorrhea, cough, N/V/D

Past medical / surgical / social history: No past medical history or prior surgery. Pt is a 0.5ppd smoker.

Scenario #3: Fall

Nurse: "Hey Doctor, we have a 75 y/o male coming from home after a fall on Coumadin."

Doctor: "Alright, we'll go right in."

(Doctor goes in room)

Doctor: "Hello, Mr. Smith, I heard you fell today. Are you on Coumadin?"

Patient: "Yes, for my a-fib."

Doctor: "Alright, when is the last time you had your INR checked?"

Patient: "Yesterday, I think it was a 2.1."

Doctor: "Tell me about your fall."

Patient: "I was in the kitchen getting something out of the cupboard and I must have lost my balance and I fell backwards and hit my head."

Doctor: "Alright, I'm going to order a head CT right away. When you take Coumadin it makes your blood thin so you have a higher chance of bleeding internally. I want to recheck your INR and make sure you aren't bleeding inside your head since you hit it. Now let's talk more about the fall. Did you lose consciousness?"

Patient: "No, I don't think so."

Doctor: "Alright good. Before you fell did you feel any chest palpitations, dizziness or shortness of breath?"

Patient: "I guess I did feel a little dizzy before I fell."

Doctor: "Were you lightheaded, or was the room spinning?"

Patient: "More lightheaded."

Doctor: "Have you had any recent fevers, chills, cough, nausea, vomiting or diarrhea?"

Patient: "I have had some diarrhea, I think I ate some bad food when we went out to eat."

Doctor: "Have you noticed your stools being black or tarry? Or has there been any blood in them?"

Patient: "No, sir. Just loose stool."

Doctor: "How many episodes of diarrhea have you had in the past day?"

Patient: "Oh, quite a few, at least 8 or 10."

Doctor: "Alright, we'll have to get some fluids in you. I suspect you are dehydrated from the diarrhea and this led to your fall. Are you in pain anywhere else?"

Patient: "No, just the back of my head."

Doctor: "OK, what other medical problems do you have besides the a-fib?"

Patient: "Well I have diabetes and high blood pressure. I had a heart attack back in 2006 and they put a stent in then."

Doctor: "Have you had any surgeries besides the stent?"

Patient: "Yes. I've had back surgery, my tonsils are out, appendix was taken out when I was a kid."

Doctor: "Alright, were you ever a smoker?"

Patient: "Yes, I smoked, quit about 8 years ago."

Doctor: "Alright, we'll get those labs and tests done. I'll be back in once I have some results."

CC: _____

HPI: _____

_____

_____

_____

_____

ROS: _____

_____

_____

_____

_____

Past medical / surgical / social history:_____

_____

_____

CC: Fall

HPI: 75 y/o male presents to ED s/p fall, on Coumadin, now c/o head pain. Pt was in the kitchen when he had an episode of dizziness described as "lightheadedness" which caused him to fall backwards and hit the back of his head on the tile floor. Pt denies LOC and was able to ambulate without complication immediately following the fall. For the past day pt has had 8-10 episodes of diarrhea. Denies hematochezia, melena, cough, SOB, chest pain, palpitations, N/V, fever or chills. Pt had INR checked 1 day which was reportedly 2.1.

ROS: Positive for dizziness, dizziness, diarrhea. Negative for melena, hematochezia, N/V, abdominal pain, chest pain, SOB, cough, fevers, chills.

Past medical / surgical / social history: Past medical: a-fib, MI, DM, HTN. Past surgical: stents (5 years ago), tonsillectomy, appendectomy. Pt is a former smoker, quit for 8 years.

Scenario #4: Altered Mental Status (AMS)

Nurse: "Doctor, this woman is coming in from a nursing home. The staff went in to her room this morning around 6 AM and found her less responsive than usual. She had a left facial droop and left arm weakness. I started the stroke scale."

Doctor: "When was she last seen at her baseline?"

Nurse: "They said around 10 PM last night"

Doctor: "Alright, then we aren't sure of the onset of her symptoms, this means she isn't a tPA candidate. What is her baseline?"

Nurse: "Well, they said she has severe dementia, and is A&O x 2 at best. She normally knows her name and where she is. We haven't been able to get any other information from her. The clerk is working on getting her health records sent over."

Doctor: "Alright, lets get a head CT and some labs and go from there. Do we know her code status?"

Nurse: "No, but her daughter who is the DPOA is on her way."

CC: _____

HPI: _____

_____

_____

_____

_____

_____

ROS: _____

_____

_____

_____

_____

Past medical / surgical / social history:_____

_____

_____

CC: Altered Mental Status

HPI: 86 y/o female with a past medical history of dementia presents to emergency with altered mental status. Around 6 AM this morning at the patient's ECF, staff found the patient less responsive than baseline. At this time, staff noticed left facial droop. Last time patient was seen at baseline was 10pm last night. EMS reports pt was noted to have left upper extremity weakness. No fall, headache, dizziness, chest pain, abdominal pain, nausea, vomiting, diarrhea, urinary symptoms, fever or chills. No other complaints or modifying factors at this time.

ROS: AMS, facial droop, weakness. Unable to be obtained due to patient's dementia.

Past-medical / surgical / social history: Past medical: dementia. Past surgical: Unable to obtain due to pt's mental status. Social: Pt is a nursing home resident.

**In a situation like this, if old records are available you can look back to obtain a better past medical history. This information may also be helpful to the physician.

Scenario #5: Ankle Injury

Doctor: "What brings you in today?"

Mother: "She was at soccer practice and she tripped and fell. She started crying immediately and won't put weight on her left ankle."

Doctor: "Ok, where is your pain at?"

Patient: "On the right on the side of my ankle."

Doctor: "Alright. It is pretty swollen and black and blue. Did you hurt anything else when you fell?"

Patient: "No."

Doctor: "OK, can you feel when I touch your toes and foot?"

Patient: "Yes."

Doctor: "Alright, lets get some x-rays. I think that might be broken. Mom, does she have any medical problems or allergies?"

Mother: "No, none that we know of."

Doctor: "OK. Would she like some ibuprofen for the pain?"

Mother: "Well, I gave her some before we came in."

Doctor: "Alright, we'll hold of on any more then."

CC: _____

HPI: _____

_____

_____

_____

_____

ROS: _____

_____

_____

_____

_____

Past medical / surgical / social history:_____

_____

_____

CC: Ankle injury

HPI: 8 y/o female with no significant past medical history who presents to emergency with left ankle pain. The patient was at soccer practice PTA when she tripped and fell injuring her left ankle. She cannot bear weight on the joint and states her pain is on the medial side of her left ankle. No numbness or tingling in the extremity. No other injuries or complaints at this time.

ROS: Positive for left ankle pain. Negative for other injury, change in sensation.

Past medical / surgical / social history: No prior medical or surgical history.

Scenario #6: Cough

Doctor: "Hello, Sir. What brings you in today?"

Patient: "I've had this cough for the past 5 days and it seems to be getting worse."

Doctor: "Is it a dry cough? Or are you bringing anything up?"

Patient: "I've been coughing up phlegm, its kind of greenish."

Doctor: "So you've had this cough for the past 5 days, what made you decide to come in today?"

Patient: "Well, it just seems like its been getting harder to breath and my chest feels really tight."

Doctor: "Have you had any fevers?"

Patient: "I haven't checked but I have had chills and sweats."

Doctor: "Alright, have you coughed up any blood?"

Patient: "No."

Doctor: "Any recent nausea, vomiting or diarrhea?"

Patient: "No."

Doctor: "How about any leg swelling or rash?"

Patient: "No."

Doctor: "Do you smoke?"

Patient: "Yeah."

Doctor: "How much?"

Patient: "About a pack per day since I was 18."

Doctor: "Do you have any medical problems?"

Patient: "Nope."

Doctor: "Any previous surgeries?"

Patient: "Just my back. I had a laminectomy."

Doctor: "Alright, well I suspect you may have a pneumonia. I'm going to do an exam and then we'll get a chest x-ray. I'm going to have the nurse get some blood cultures to make sure the infection hasn't spread into your blood."

CC: _____

HPI: _____

_____

_____

_____

_____

_____

ROS: _____

_____

_____

_____

_____

Past medical / surgical / social history:_____

_____

_____

CC: Cough

HPI: 58 y/o male presents to ED c/o cough productive of greenish sputum x 5 days with associated chest "tightness" and progressively worsening dyspnea. Pt also reports subjective fever with chills and sweats. Denies hemoptysis, nausea, vomiting, diarrhea, edema, rash. Pt is a 1ppd smoker x 40 years.

ROS: Positive for: cough, chest tightness, dyspnea, green sputum, chills, sweats and fever
Negative for: hemoptysis, N/V/D, edema, rash

Past medical / surgical / social history: none; surg: laminectomy soc: smoke 1ppd x 40 years

Scenario #7: Leg Ulcer

Doctor: "Hello, ma'am. What brings you in today?"

Patient: "I have this sore on my leg that I noticed 2 days ago. I took some clindamycin but it didn't go away so I came in."

Doctor: "Where did you get the clindamycin?"

Patient: "I had it leftover from last year when I had bronchitis."

Doctor: "Alright, well have you had any other symptoms? Fever, sweats, chills, nausea, vomiting, diarrhea, abdominal pain?"

Patient: "Nope, I have been healthy."

Doctor: "How about abdominal pain or headache?"

Patient: "No."

Doctor: "Any problems with urination? Pain or burning? Blood in your urine?"

Patient: "No."

Doctor: "Alright, do you have any medical problems?"

Patient: "I have diabetes and high blood pressure."

Doctor: "Are you on insulin?"

Patient: "Yes, I am. And I check my sugar everyday."

Doctor: "How have your sugars been?"

Patient: "In the right range, nothing too high or low."

Doctor: "Alright good. Have you missed any doses of your insulin?"

Patient: "No, I have not."

Doctor: "Good. Have you had any surgeries in the past?"

Patient: "I had a knee replacement on the right, and a C-section way back when I had my daughter."

Doctor: "Do you smoke or drink?"

Patient: "No."

Doctor: "Alright good, are you working now?"

Patient: "No, I am retired. I used to be a teacher."

Doctor: "Alright, well this looks like it's pretty deep, and with your history of diabetes I think I'd like to bring you in to the hospital overnight to get some IV antibiotics. I'm also going to have the nurse get some blood cultures to make sure there isn't any infection that has spread there."

CC: _____

HPI: _____

_____

_____

_____

_____

_____

ROS: _____

_____

_____

_____

_____

Past medical / surgical / social history:_____

_____

_____

CC: Leg Ulcer

HPI: 67 y/o female with h/o HTN, IDDM presents to ED c/o LLE ulcer x 2 days. Pt first noticed the ulcer 2 days ago on her left lateral calf. At that time she took some Clindamycin that she had left over from a previous infection, but has not seen any improvement . She states her DM has been well controlled and has not missed any of her insulin doses. Denies fever, chills, dizziness, headache, hematuria, dysuria, abdominal pain, N/V/D.

ROS: Leg ulcer with surrounding erythema

Negative for: fever, sweats, chills, N/V/D, dizziness, abdominal pain, headache, hematuria, dysuria

Past med/surg/soc: Med: IDDM, HTN. Surg: right knee replacement, c-section. Social: never smoker, does not drink, retired

Scenario #8: Unresponsive

EMS: "Patient is a 71 year old male who was found by his daughter unresponsive in the pool. Patient has a past medical history of hypertension and previous MI with stent placement."

Doctor: "How long was he unresponsive?"

EMS: "We don't know. He was swimming in the pool by himself and the daughter found him belly down in the pool. A bystander was there who knew CPR. He started CPR while the daughter called us. We got the call at 1:00 pm and arrived on the scene at 1:05 pm."

Doctor: "Did you get a reading on the EKG at any time?"

EMS: "No. The patient has been in asystole the entire time."

Doctor: "Is family on the way?"

EMS: "Yes. The daughter was pulling in right behind us."

CC: _____

HPI: _____

_____

_____

_____

_____

ROS: _____

_____

_____

_____

_____

Past medical / surgical / social history:_____

_____

_____

CC: Unresponsive

HPI: Pt is a 71 year old male with a past medical history of hypertension, MI and stent placement who presents to emergency unresponsive. He was swimming alone in his pool when his daughter found him unresponsive, belly-down in the pool. A bystander helped pull the patient out of the pool and began CPR. CPR was done for approximately 20 minutes prior to EMS arrival. Pt has remained in asystole per EMS report.

ROS: Unable to be obtained due to patient unresponsive.

Past medical / surgical / social history: hypertension, MI and stent placement

Scenario #9: Flank Pain

Doctor: "Hello sir, what brings you in today?"

Patient: "I am so uncomfortable. I have a lot of pain in the middle of my back on the right side."

Doctor: "When did the pain start?"

Patient: "3 hours ago and it hasn't let up since. It feels like there is a knife in my back and it's getting worse!"

Doctor: "Are you nauseous?"

Patient: "Nauseous, yes. But I haven't thrown up."

Doctor: "Do you have any urinary symptoms, burning with urination, urinating more frequently?"

Patient: "Burning, but I haven't been going more frequently."

Doctor: "Any blood?"

Patient: "No. Ah it hurts so bad! Please give me medicine."

Doctor: "I will. Have you ever had a kidney stone before?"

Patient: "No. Never."

Doctor: "Any medical problems?"

Patient: "No."

Doctor: "Well I think you might have one. I am going to order some pain medicine and send you off to CT."

CC: _____

HPI: _____

_____

_____

_____

_____

ROS: _____

_____

_____

_____

_____

Past medical / surgical / social history:_____

_____

_____

CC: Right Flank Pain

HPI: Pt is a 25 year old male with no significant past medical history who presents to emergency with right sided flank pain. 3 hours PTA the patient developed right sided flank pain that has increased since onset and is described as a stabbing pain. Pt has associated nausea and dysuria with no vomiting, hematuria or urinary frequency. No dizziness, chest pain, abdominal pain, bowel symptoms, fever or chills. No other complaints or modifying factors at this time.

ROS: Nausea and dysuria. Negative for vomiting, hematuria, urinary frequency, dizziness, chest pain, abdominal pain, bowel symptoms, fever or chills.

Past medical / surgical / social history: No significant past medical history.

Scenario #10: Vaginal Bleeding

Doctor: "Hello ma'am. What brings you to emergency today?"

Patient: "Well. I am currently 8 weeks pregnant with my first child and I started bleeding last night."

Doctor: "How much blood have you noticed?"

Patient: "I have been soaking one pad every hour."

Doctor: "That is a lot of blood. Do you feel light headed at all?"

Patient: "No. Not at all."

Doctor: "Alright. Do you have any abdominal pain?"

Patient: "Cramping in the lower part."

Doctor: "But no pain?"

Patient: "No. It just feels like menstrual cramping."

Doctor: "Have you had a check up for this pregnancy yet?"

Patient: "Yes. I had my first ultrasound 6 weeks ago that was normal."

Doctor: "When was your last menstrual period?"

Patient: "About 11 weeks ago now."

Doctor: "Any nausea, vomiting, urinary symptoms?"

Patient: "No. Everything else is fine. Just the bleeding and cramping."

Doctor: "Any past medical history?"

Patient: "No."

Doctor: "Do you smoke?"

Patient: "No."

Doctor: "Drink?"

Patient: "No."

Doctor: "Okay. We are going to order an ultrasound and see what is going on."

CC: _____

HPI: _____

_____

_____

_____

_____

_____

ROS: _____

_____

_____

_____

_____

Past medical / surgical / social history:_____

_____

_____

CC: Vaginal Bleeding

HPI: Pt is a 29 year old female (G0P1A0) with no past medical history presents to emergency complaining of vaginal bleeding. Last night the patient began bleeding vaginally and reports soaking one pad per hour since onset. Pt is currently 8 weeks pregnant and had a normal ultrasound at 6 weeks confirming the pregnancy. Bleeding is associated with lower abdominal cramping similar to menstrual cramps per patient. Pt denies any abdominal pain. LMP was 11 weeks ago.

ROS: No dizziness, chest pain, nausea, vomiting, urinary or bowel symptoms, fever or chills. No other complaints or modifying factors at this time.

Past medical / surgical / social history: Ptp has no past medical history, non-smoker, denies alcohol use.

Scenario #11: Drug Overdose

EMS: "Patient is a known heroin addict. His mom told us that today he was having a bad day. She heard a loud thud on the patient's bedroom floor and she ran upstairs to see what happened. She found the patient with a syringe on the bed and she immediately called 911."

Doctor: "Was he responsive?"

EMS: "The mother said she was shouting his name and he wasn't responding, but when we got there he was just mumbling a bunch of stuff like he is now. He does respond and look at you if you yell his name loudly."

Doctor: "Does she know if he had anything else?"

EMS: "Mom says there was a fifth of Jack in the patient's room so she isn't sure if he also had alcohol. But she confirms heroin because she found more in the patient's bedroom."

Doctor: "Alright. Any past medical history?"

EMS: "Just the heroin use. Nothing else."

CC: _____

HPI: _____

_____

_____

_____

_____

ROS: _____

_____

_____

_____

_____

Past medical / surgical / social history:_____

_____

_____

CC: Drug Overdose

HPI: Pt is a 23 year old male with a past medical history significant for heroin abuse presents to emergency after a drug overdose. Per mother, the patient was having a bad day and was upstairs in his bedroom when she heard a loud thud on the floor. She ran upstairs and found the patient unresponsive with a heroin syringe on his bed. EMS responded and found the patient sitting up mumbling and able to respond to loud stimuli. Mother states that there was alcohol present in the patient's bedroom and she is unsure if the patient consumed any prior to this incident. No modifying factors at this time.

ROS: Unable to obtain due to patient's current condition.

Past medical / surgical / social history: Past medical history significant for heroin abuse.

Scenario #12: Suicide Attempt

Doctor: "So, tell me what happened tonight?"

Patient: "Yesterday was the one year anniversary of my dad's passing and I have been really depressed the whole week."

Doctor: "I'm sorry for your loss."

Patient: "Thanks. It has been really hard and I felt like I had to come here or something might happen."

Doctor: "What would happen?"

Patient: "I don't know. I might do something."

Doctor: "We're you thinking of harming yourself?"

Patient: "Kinda."

Doctor: "How?"

Patient: "I dunno exactly how, but I just thought if I end my life then I could see my dad again."

Doctor: "You never had an actual plan?"

Patient: "No. No actual plans. Just ideas running through my head."

Doctor: "Are you hearing voices?"

Patient: "No."

Doctor: "Have you used any drugs tonight? Or Alcohol?"

Patient: "No. Never do drugs. Alcohol occasionally but not this week."

Doctor: "Do you feel like harming anyone else?"

Patient: "Never. I would never want to harm anyone else because I know how miserable I am without my father."

Doctor: "Okay. Any past medical history?"

Patient: "I have struggled with depression before, but I was never put on medication for it. And no other actual medical problems. I have been lucky."

Doctor: "Alright. In the emergency room we have to complete basic lab work just to make sure you are medically cleared. But I am also going to have the social worker come in to talk to you about everything and hopefully she can get you grief counseling."

CC: _____

HPI: _____

_____

_____

_____

_____

ROS: _____

_____

_____

_____

_____

Past medical / surgical / social history: _____

_____

_____

CC: Suicidal Ideation

HPI: Pt is a 30 year old female with a past medical history for depression presents to emergency with suicidal ideation. Yesterday was the anniversary of her father passing away and the patient states she has been in a depressed state all week. She states she came to the ER because "she had to come here or something might happen. She might do something". She states she does not have an exact plan on how to end her life. No homicidal ideation. No hallucinations. No drug or alcohol use. No other medical complaints at this time.

ROS: Suicidal Ideation

Past medical / surgical / social history: Past medical history for depression.

16

STUDY GUIDES AND QUIZZES

The following pages contain the study guides for the quizzes that you will be required to complete and pass during your training shifts. To pass a quiz you must obtain a score of 90% or higher.

Quiz #1 Study Guide

1. Know what elements go in each element of the chart. Know the elements of the HPI. Know 3 types of radiology tests. Know what the following labs are for: LFT, Troponin, BHCG. Know all common procedures done in the ED and why they are performed.
2. Know the following terms for spelling and definitions: nephrolithiasis, atrial fibrillation, stenosis, hemotympanum, syncope, hemorrhage, rticarial, vertigo, Parethesia, tinnitus
3. Know the following abbreviations: ASA, TID, Abx, SOB, XR
4. Know the following medications (spelling and general use): Toradol, Prednisone, Hydrochlorothiazide, Omeprazole, Ativan

Quiz #2 Study Guide

1. Practice HPI writing
2. Know following terms (definitions and spelling): tachypnea, angina, icterus, menorrhagia, jaundice, cachectic, capillary refill, hyperkalemia, petechial, ascites
3. Know abbreviations: AAA, CAD, DTR, TIA, SVT
4. Know meds (spelling and general use): Depakote, Warfarin, Labetalol, Fluorescein, Haldol

Quiz #3 Study Guide

1. Know the coding elements (memorize table)
2. Know terms (spelling and definitions): bruit, photophobia, hypertension, hemoptysis, epistaxis, melena, emesis, hemorrhoids, somnolent, myocardial infarction
3. Know abbreviations: appy, fx, NPO, UE, UTI

4.   Know meds: flagyl, metoprolol, Compazine, clindamycin, versed

Quiz #4 Study Guide

1. Know critical charting elements for each common case.
2. Know terms: aneurysm, cardiomyopathy, nares, paronychia, dehiscense, hemoptysis, COPD, lymphadenopathy, ischemia, epistaxis
3. Know abbreviations: AMS, r/o, PE, OM, GSW
4. Know meds: Acetaminophen, Zofran, Dilantin, Albuterol, Phenergan

Quiz #5 Study Guide

1.   Terms: atherosclerosis, sputum, diaphoresis, dyspnea, cardiomyopathy, nystagmus, psychosis, leukocytosis, diplopia, malocclusion, malleolus, diverticulosis, STEMI, amenorrhea, arthralgia, arrhythmia, ascites, cholelithiasis, hypoxia, deep vein thrombosis
2.   Abbreviations: AMA, BM, CVA, VS, PRN, Rx, HA, IDDM, LLQ, MI
3.   Meds: Amoxicillin, Klonopin, Lasix, Lidocaine, Levaquin

Quiz #6 Study Guide

1. Terms: Cardiomegaly, dyspnea, psoriasis, anasarca, prostatitis, Cerumen, cholecystitis, dyspepsia, amenorrhea, nystagmus, pneumothorax, coronary artery disease, hyperlipidemia, dysmenorrhea, menorrhagia, dehiscence, erythema, ecchymosis, febrile, sepsis
2. Abbreviations: BP, WPW, PO, CA, WNL, PCP, DVT, PERRLA, NSR
3. Meds: Azithromycin, Ceftriaxone, Coumadin, Atenolol, Diltiazem

Quiz #7 Study Guide

1. Terms: atelectasis, ventricular hypertrophy, palpitations, rhinorrhea, hematemesis, dyspareunia, hyperkalemia, hematochezia, cholecystectomy, hypernatremia, cachectic, pyelonephritis, emaciated, rhabdomyolysis, dysphagia, myalgia, aphasia, debridement, diaphoresis, dysuria, hematuria, Parethesia, torsion, cellulitis

2. Abbreviations: CHF, DKA, DM, TM, ESRD, CTA, ETOH, K, NAD, HTN
3. Meds: Rocephin, Vancomycin, Solumedrol, Plavix, Simvastatin

Quiz 1

Elements of a Chart

S: The _____ part of the note. This is the part told from _____'s perspective. It includes the: _____, _____, _____.

    Details that should be included in the HPI (list at least 5 for full credit)

    1. _____

    2. _____

    3. _____

    4. _____

    5. _____

O: The _____ part of the note. This is the part told from _____'s perspective. It includes the: _____, _____, _____.

    List 3 types of radiology tests:

    1. _____

    2. _____

    3. _____

List 3 common lab tests and what they are used for:

1. LFTs :_____

2. Troponin: _____

3. BHCG: _____

A: _____.

P: _____.

This section is the doctor's explanation of the patient and the plan for treatment:_____

Common procedure to treat an abscess: _____

Common procedure to obtain CSF: _____

Common procedure performed in order to obtain long term IV access or give certain medications: _____

Vocabulary

Spelling:
1.   _____

2.   _____

3.   _____

4. _____

5. _____

Definitions:

1._____

2._____

3._____

4._____

5._____

Abbreviations:

1. _____

2. _____

3. _____

4. _____

5. _____

Medications:

1. _____

2. _____

3. _____

4. _____

5. _____

Quiz 2

HPI: Trainer will read a case to you. While you are listening, write an HPI. Include as many elements as you hear. There will be a total of 8. You will receive 0.5 pts off for each missed element. This portion counts for a total of 4pts.

_____

_____

_____

_____

_____

_____

_____

_____

_____

_____

Vocabulary

Spelling:

1. _____

2. _____

3. _____

4. _____

5. _____

Definitions:

6._____

7._____

8._____

9._____

10._____

Abbreviations: 2. _____

1. _____   3. _____

4. _____

5. _____

Medications:

1. _____

2. _____

3. _____

4. _____

5. _____

Quiz 3

Coding elements

1.   How many elements are needed in a level 5 HPI? _____

2.   How many elements are needed in a level 3 ROS? _____

3.   How many elements are needed in a level 3 physical exam? _____

4.   How many elements are needed in a level 5 physical exam? _____

5.   How many elements are needed in a level 3 HPI? _____

6.   How many elements are needed in the past history section in a level 3 chart?
_____, a level 5? _____.

Vocabulary

Spelling:

1.   _____

2.   _____

3.   _____

4.   _____

5.   _____

Definitions:

1._____

2._____

3._____

4._____

5._____

Abbreviations:

1. _____

2. _____

3. _____

4. _____

5. _____

Medications:

1. _____

2. _____

3. _____

4. _____

5. _____

Quiz 4

1.   List a critical element to chart for a chest pain:

2.   List critical elements to chart for a MHE:

3.   List critical elements to chart for a TIA/CVA:

4.   List elements to chart for a MVA:

Vocabulary

Spelling:

1.   _____

2.   _____

3.   _____

4.   _____

5.   _____

Definitions:

1.   _____

2.   _____

3.   _____

4. _____

5. _____

Medications:

1. _____

2. _____

Abbreviations:

3. _____

1. _____

4. _____

2. _____

5. _____

3. _____

4. _____

5. _____

Vocabulary

Spelling:

1. _____

2. _____

3. _____

4. _____

5. _____

6. _____

7. _____

8. _____

9. _____

10. _____

Definitions:

1._____

2._____

3._____

4._____

5._____

6._____

7._____

8._____

9._____

10._____

Abbreviations:

1. _____   6. _____

2. _____   7. _____

3. _____   8. _____

4. _____   9. _____

5. _____   10. _____

Quiz 6

Vocabulary

Spelling:

1. _____   6. _____

2. _____   7. _____

3. _____   8. _____

4. _____   9. _____

5. _____   10. _____

Definitions:

1._____

2._____

3._____

4._____

5._____

6._____

7._____

8._____

9._____

10._____

Abbreviations:

1._____   6._____

2._____   7._____

3._____   8._____

4._____   9._____

5._____   10._____

Quiz 7

Vocabulary

Spelling:

1. _____

2. _____

3. _____

4. _____

5. _____

6. _____

7. _____

8. _____

9. _____

10. _____

Definitions:

1. _____

2. _____

3. _____

4. _____

5. _____

6. _____

7. _____

8._____

9._____

10._____

Abbreviations:

1. _____   6. _____

2. _____   7. _____

3. _____   8. _____

4. _____   9. _____

5. _____   10. _____

Bibliography

Advisory Board Company, The. (1999). Practice #3: Charting Scribe. Liberating Physician Time , 59-81.

American College of Emergency Physicians. (2012). Physician Quality Reporting System FAQ. Retrieved 01 15, 2012, from the American College of Emergency Physicians: http://www.acep.org/content.aspx?id=30492

Joint Commission, The. (2011). Specifications Manual for National Hospital Inpatient Quality Measures. Retreived 01 15, 2012, from The Joint Commission: http://www.jointcommission.org/specifications_manual_for_national_hospital_inpatient_quality_measures/

Joint Commission, The. (2010, 10 22). Core Measure Sets. Retreived 01 15, 2012, from The Joint Commission: http://www.jointcommission.org/core_measure_set/

U.S. Department of Health and Human Services. (2012). Health Information Privacy. Retrieved 01 15, 2012, from U.S. Department of Health and Human Services: http://www.hhs.gov/ocr/privacy/

17880403R00117

Made in the USA
Lexington, KY
02 October 2012